My Bump & Me

My Bump & Me

Myleene
Klass

**From morning sickness to motherhood –
an honest diary of my pregnancy**

Selected and edited by Nicole Lampert

Virgin
BOOKS

To yummy mummies everywhere: you are all goddesses in my eyes.
To my own mum for the compassion and love she taught and gave
me. And to my baby girl, Ava. Thank you for choosing me to be your
mama. The second I held you, my heart was yours.

Published by Virgin Books 2009
2 4 6 8 10 9 7 5 3

Copyright © Myleene Klass 2008

Myleene Klass has asserted her right under the Copyright, Designs
and Patents Act 1988 to be identified as the author of this work

First published in Great Britain in 2008 by Virgin Books
Random House, 20 Vauxhall Bridge Road, London SW1V 2SA

www.virginbooks.com
www.rbooks.co.uk

Addresses for companies within The Random House Group Limited can be found at:
www.randomhouse.co.uk/offices.htm

The Random House Group Limited Reg. No. 954009

A CIP catalogue record for this book
is available from the British Library

ISBN 9780753515563

The Random House Group Limited supports The Forest Stewardship Council [FSC], the
leading international forest certification organisation. All our titles that are printed on
Greenpeace approved FSC certified paper carry the FSC logo.
Our paper procurement policy can be found at www.rbooks.co.uk/environment

Printed and bound in Great Britain by
CPI Bookmarque, Croydon, CR0 4TD

All photographs courtesy of Myleene Klass/Stuart White unless otherwise stated

Contents

✳❋✳

Introduction

I always imagined the day I would tell my beloved we were expecting our first child. There would be a romantic dinner. We would have been laughing all night. We would be looking at each other lovingly. Then I would calmly present him with a pair of Manchester United bootees as I told him, 'We're having a baby, darling.'

Fast-forward to January 2007 and my fiancé Gray and I had spent another night arguing. We had hardly seen each other since I had come out of the *I'm A Celebrity* jungle and our New Year's holiday had been hijacked by both our families. As well as being rushed off my feet with work I felt constantly sick and teary. I was in such a perpetual bad mood that Gray was calling me a witch.

It was close to midnight and I was exhausted. My boobs were hurting like mad and I couldn't work out why I was feeling so strange. I can't say how or why – and really I should have spotted the symptoms some days before – but I suddenly realised what was wrong with me. I told Gray I needed a pregnancy test straightaway.

We hadn't been trying for a baby and it was the last thing either of us ever expected.

But from that moment on I became a different person. I now had a baby inside me to look after – and I didn't know how on earth to go about it.

I read lots of books but found them either too fluffy or too technical. Most of them terrified me. I wanted answers but all I got were lists of 'don't do this' and 'don't do that'. All they made me realise was that I had supposedly done everything wrong.

None seemed to relate to how I was feeling. I was so sick, I was so tired, I was so teary. I felt so isolated and my pregnancy seemed so different to how I always saw it portrayed in the movies or in interviews with celebrities.

So if you are a woman who has become someone she can hardly recognise, who has cried over the nursery curtains being the wrong colour or because your partner forgot to put a kiss at the end of his text message, this book is for you. I want you to know that you are not alone.

This book tells the truth about pregnancy. The highs and the lows. And the tears, oh yes, the tears.

I used to consider myself a strong and resilient girl. I have got through plenty of heartache in my time and have happily jumped out of planes and been in other extreme situations. But being pregnant meant I would quiver at the slightest setback. I cried more in the nine months I was pregnant than I have in my entire lifetime.

Being pregnant made me panic over eating peanut butter and whether I could walk through airport security scanners.

I forgot the names of some of the most famous (and gorgeous) men in the world and made up words on live television because my memory got so bad.

I rowed with my beloved Gray (Graham Quinn), a security guard who has been my partner for the last six years, more times than I care to remember.

And at the end of my journey, as I became a mother, I realised that I would never go back to being the woman I once was.

As well as detailing exactly what I went through I have included facts about what is happening to you and your baby each week. I used to love reading these in books as it is amazing to think about the changes going on in your tummy every week.

I don't, however, claim to be a doctor and this is not a very medical pregnancy book. I have written a list at the end of ones that I found useful for all those fears you are likely to get.

This diary is based on real diaries that Gray and I started keeping once we discovered I was pregnant. Gray saw things in such a different way from me that it was an eye-opener to read his entries. I feel guilty for the way I sometimes behaved towards him but I couldn't control my hormones – they changed me so much I felt like I'd had a lobotomy.

So along with chapters about my pregnancy journey I have included his thoughts, hopes and comments too. Sometimes it is easy to forget that the daddy is going through pregnancy too – even if that just means being at the end of your foul moods and being pushed out of bed by your big tummy and snoring.

Pregnancy and becoming a mummy haven't just made me appreciate Gray. They have made me realise how incredible my own mother is, and how amazing all my mummy friends are.

Once you fall pregnant you become part of a club. It's a club where you stop putting yourself first – everything becomes about the baby, including the awe-inspiring changes your body goes through. It's a club where you often struggle to cope. And it's a club in which you learn just how much you can love another being.

If you are reading this because you are pregnant, welcome to the best club in the world. I hope this book makes you realise you are not alone in all your hormonal behaviour, 'baby brain' is a common affliction and the sheer worry that comes during your pregnancy is normal.

My pregnancy was an often emotional and sometimes difficult journey but the reward was the best thing I have ever known.

Myleene

PS The weekly sidebars in this book are based only on average measurements. All babies develop differently in the womb . . . so that's one less thing to worry about!

Weeks 1 & 2

The Jungle Weeks – My Body Prepared to Make a Baby

✳❇✳

I have promised to tell you the truth about pregnancy so I will start with a confession: getting pregnant was an accident. A gorgeously happy accident.

When I decided to go into the Australian rainforest for *I'm A Celebrity . . . Get Me Out of Here!* the idea of having a baby was, in fact, the last thing on my mind.

Although I have never wanted to be one of those women who say, 'I'll just see where my career takes me this year,' only to find they are nearly fifty and unable to conceive, I was still only 28 and felt like I had some time left on the biological clock.

I also felt that, struggling as I was to look after myself, I wasn't sure I was ready to be a mother just yet.

My partner Gray, however, was desperate to be a dad. He was a bit older – 33 – and lots of his friends had children and he was beginning to feel like he was missing out.

I had been using a contraceptive injection for years but came off it about a year before I went into the jungle to give my body a break. My periods still hadn't regulated and, although we used protection occasionally, I was convinced there would not be much chance of me being fertile until everything was back in order.

I admit that I feel like a silly seventeen-year-old now when I think about how naïve we were being about contraception.

But in my defence, m'lord, a friend who had also been on the same injection took more than eighteen months to get pregnant and I have had so many friends who have had problems conceiving that I was sure I would have to wait another six months before I needed to even think about contraception.

I guess that buried deep in my mind was also the thought that if I were to fall pregnant it would not be the end of the world. Gray and I had been together for more than six years and were engaged to be married. Our plan had always been to start a family one day.

But we certainly were not expecting it to be on the day I came out of the jungle.

I had agreed to go on *I'm A Celebrity* after turning it down for three previous years. I knew that being on the show was either going to be the death knell of my career or mean that I was suddenly going to be a lot busier. I was doing it partly to test myself, partly to get a break from work and partly (yes, I know it's a cliché) to show the public the 'real' me.

Up until I went into the jungle, I was still best known as the girl who had been in Hear'Say. Although I had been working as a classical musician, a DJ and a television presenter on CD:UK, I knew that in order to give my career a real kick-start I needed to do something mainstream like *I'm A Celebrity*.

So I guess I can't blame anyone but myself that I became famous for having showers in my white bikini while on the show. In all honesty I never realised the producers were making such a big deal of my showers – after all, I wasn't showering any more than the next person! I was much more proud of my DIY achievements like building the camp a table and a broomstick – but to my disappointment nobody made a fuss of those.

Still, I certainly can't complain – going on the show has meant I'm now busier than I have ever been before. And, more importantly, it provided the perfect environment to prepare my body for pregnancy.

You won't find jumping out of planes, showering with spiders, bathing with eels, not to mention ducking out of the way of celebrity rows, advised in most pregnancy manuals. But in a strange sort of way, being in the *I'm A Celebrity* jungle was the textbook environment for the pre-conception of my baby.

Advice for women wanting to get pregnant includes getting fit, detoxing, eating healthily and trying to stay relaxed. And in the rainforest, the hikes, the physical activities, the meagre alcohol allowance and the protein-orientated meals meant that I was in the best physical condition of my life. I was away from all the stresses of modern-day living, so was feeling more relaxed and liberated than I had ever done before. And I was well rested because I was sleeping when it got dark.

I adored living at one with nature – even the spiders and bugs didn't bother me – but I wasn't to know nature was planning a little surprise for me.

What's happening to your body – Weeks 1 and 2

The forty weeks of pregnancy are dated from two weeks before your baby has actually been conceived. The first day is the start of your period when the lining of your womb is shed, giving it a 'spring-clean' in preparation for the arrival of a fertilised egg. Ovulation normally occurs on the last day of the second week when one (or occasionally more) of the eggs you were born with is released into the Fallopian tube in preparation for fertilisation. You can often tell you are ovulating as your body produces extra vaginal mucus.

Week 3

The Week in Which Our Baby Was Conceived

Gray and I had just one hour to spend together from the time I left the jungle before I had to start work again and we were determined to use it properly.

I was busy getting showered and putting my make-up on ahead of having to do a round of interviews and photoshoots when Gray followed me into the bathroom. There were dozens of journalists, television executives and press officers milling about nearby but, as it had been almost two months since we had any time together, we decided to seize our moment.

Gray was not even supposed to be in Australia as he was due to be working on a band's tour. I was devastated because I had missed him so much and was very emotional when I left the jungle thinking he was not going to be there.

But then, when all the filming was finished and I crossed that famous bridge, I saw him. It was a proper Mills & Boon moment. We went running into each other's arms and Gray told me how much he had missed me and how he wanted us to get our act together and get married.

We first met when Gray was working as a bodyguard for Hear'Say. We did not get a great impression of each other to begin with – I thought he was really rude while he was annoyed that I had once stolen his dinner. But when he joined the band on our tour I became impressed at the way he was so different to all the other 'yes men' around us. He was refreshing because he wasn't afraid to tell us when we were being out of order.

Every evening, it was Gray's job to drop off all the stuff we had left in our dressing room into our bedrooms. We would often have a good chat and I began to realise that I had romantic feelings for him – and I was sure that he felt the same way. So one night, as he was about to leave the room, I went to give him a kiss.

It was a disaster. He moved his head away and said, 'I can't do this,' and walked out, leaving my heart on the floor. I was absolutely mortified.

We ignored each other all the next day – I was too upset to even look him in the eye – but that evening when he came to my room we had a heart-to-heart. He said he did have strong feelings for me but was worried that he would look unprofessional. He then said the sweetest thing: 'I want the fairy tale,' he told me. 'I don't want this to be just a fling.' We have been together ever since.

Although my friends have always teased us about being 'the perfect couple', you won't have to read far into this book to see that, like any couple, we are far from it. But we have been through

My tip You can get ovulation sticks, you can measure your basal temperature and you can do a dozen other things to make sure that it is the 'right time' to conceive a baby. But sometimes things cannot be planned to precision, and sometimes accidents happen.

a lot together – and that has made us stronger.

Two years ago Gray asked me to be his wife on an amazing surprise trip to Rome. Although the day he had planned had gone disastrously – I broke his treasured £500 motorcycle helmet, we got lost in the pouring rain and ran out of petrol, we were exhausted and ratty, I thought the scroll he gave me with a poem in it was a Toblerone bar! – it was also the most romantic thing to ever happen to me.

As Catholics we always meant to marry before having children and our parents had been bugging us about it for years. But our lives always seemed too busy to organise a wedding.

And following my stint in the jungle, and our little reunion afterwards, things were about to get a lot busier.

What's happening to your body – Week 3

As your egg is pushed slowly down your abdominal cavity towards your Fallopian tube by finger-like projections called fimbria, millions of sperm are swimming upwards in an attempt to be the one to fertilise it. The sperm release an enzyme that allows only one to penetrate the tough outer membrane of the egg, which then closes up. The lucky sperm carries on swimming through the egg – itself the size of a pinhead yet a hundred times bigger than the sperm – until it reaches the nucleus and the two fuse to form one cell. The sex of your baby depends on which chromosome the sperm is carrying: an X for a girl and a Y for a boy. The embryo then moves along the Fallopian tube into the uterine cavity.

Week 4

The Week When I Got My 'Period'

I had a period just before the show started, I got another one while I was in the jungle and then I had what I thought was a third a week or so after I came out.

I was used to my periods being irregular since I had come off my contraception, but this seemed mad as that meant I'd had three periods in the space of about six weeks.

The final one seemed very light – but I thought that was only down to the fact that the one in the jungle had been very heavy. I certainly felt pre-menstrual enough – but as the days went on my normal PMT got worse not better. In fact, I'd categorise those early days as being like having PMT times a hundred.

Of course, now I know that it was not a period at all – but was an early sign of pregnancy.

Around the same time I also had a medical and urine test before I started doing *The People's Quiz*. They told me one of the many things they would be able to tell was whether I was pregnant, though they didn't actually test for this and so I never found out at this stage.

I thought I had better include this information as it will help to explain why I ignored all my glaringly obvious pregnancy symptoms which had already started.

My tip Bleeding can be common in early pregnancy, especially around the time your period is due. If you have lots of pregnancy symptoms but still had some bleeding it might be worth getting yourself a test. If you are worried about bleeding in pregnancy make sure you speak to your doctor.

What's happening to your body – Week 4

You: For most women the first sign that you are pregnant is that either you have no menstrual period at all or only a very light spotting. Many of the things you normally experience before a period continue – as your breasts become more sensitive and your tummy bloated – but your body already knows it is pregnant and starts producing a hormone called hCG (human chorionic gonadotrophin). HCG is the hormone detected in pregnancy tests, which will start showing up positive around the date your period is due.

Your baby: The apple-pip-sized structure growing inside you – known as a blastocyst – is a ball of cells which will divide and develop into your baby, the placenta and the umbilical cord. It normally implants in the uterus between nine and twelve days after conception.

Week 5

The Week the Hormones Kicked in and I Started to Question My Sanity

I was convinced that Gray no longer loved me. I felt constantly sick and was arguing with everyone. My boobs felt sore, I couldn't stop crying and my face had broken out in spots. I had a raging appetite and I was exhausted. But I hadn't worked out I was pregnant – instead I and everyone around me began to question whether I was going nuts.

Hardest of all were the constant rows that started between me and Gray. They were nightly and they were horrible. We have never been a couple who really row with each other – one of us always calms things down – but now we were having screaming arguments over the most ridiculous things. It was like we hated each other.

One debate that went on and on was after the *I'm A Celebrity* wrap party when Gray decided to invite some of the people he met while I was in the jungle, plus a whole lot of strangers, back to our house for a party. I was exhausted and feeling ill and we started arguing when I said I didn't want everyone coming back to ours. The bickering continued in the car home in front of my cousin. 'Why did you have to invite so many people back ... Why are you such a killjoy ... I wouldn't have minded a few people ...

Yes, as long as they were people you wanted . . . You're so selfish . . . You're a moody cow . . .' And while my cousin went to bed, we went on at each other until the early hours of the morning. The row continued for days.

But that was not the only thing we fought over. It was always the pettiest of things – like if Gray didn't answer one of my texts all day or if I was working late and he ate dinner without me. I genuinely thought Gray had turned into the Antichrist.

Things came to a crux around New Year when we were due to have our families over. Just before our party started we had another tearful row. I remember telling Gray: 'I don't even know why we are having everyone around. There's no point – we're not talking to each other and you are just being miserable all the time.'

We tried to hide our problems at the party but everyone noticed something was wrong. Gray's sister Lisa pulled me into the wardrobe and said, 'What's wrong with you and Gray? Don't you love him any more?' My heart was racing and the tears came to my eyes. 'Of course I love him,' I sobbed. 'But I don't think he loves me.'

After they left, Gray's mother rang and said: 'I've never seen you like this, what's wrong with you and Gray? You two are normally the picture of young love.' Everybody could see there was something wrong and that we were as close to breaking up as we have ever, ever been.

And it wasn't just Gray. I was having horrible rows with my manager Jonathan Shalit. Someone at his office who worked closely with me had moved departments while I was away and I had taken it personally – to the extent that I was crying over it every day.

There was one afternoon when he had decided to take our argument out of the office – only for me to burst out crying on the street. While I was sobbing, tears running down my face,

My tip For most people the most obvious sign they are pregnant is when their period fails to show up. But, as in my case and for many others, sometimes you can get some spotting, which can confuse you. Other signs of early pregnancy include the following – you may have some, you may have them all (you poor thing) or you may have none at all:

- Changeable moods
- Sore / AGONISING boobs
- Feeling sick / being sick
- Feeling light-headed
- Needing to go to the toilet a lot
- Having a heightened sense of smell
- Craving certain foods
- Having a metallic taste in your mouth
- Being exhausted – yet having trouble sleeping

someone came up and asked for an autograph. I signed it and carried on my tearful discussion with Jonathan. Then someone else came up and asked for an autograph, which I signed in between dabbing my mascara-soaked eyes.

Concerned about my tears – and the fact that my blotchy face might not be the best look – Jonathan said to me, 'You've got to get in the car,' and that just started me off in more hysterics. 'That's just the sort of thing you would say,' I wailed at my increasingly bemused manager.

Jonathan and Gray had started to talk about what to do with me – they did not know what was wrong.

Nor did I. Part of me blamed Gray and his attitude towards me. I thought that while I was away he had reassessed everything and did not love me any more.

But I also knew that I had changed and the only thing I could put it down to was being in the rainforest. I thought – oh, the irony! – I had become so in tune with nature that I couldn't cope with the modern world.

As well as being constantly upset, I had become like a sniffer dog with smells – although most of them made me feel nauseous. I put it down to the fact that I'd had such a huge detox that my cleansed system could no longer cope with synthetic aromas. I was craving fruit and meat and in my somewhat warped reasoning this all made sense – I only wanted natural things!

I thought I had suddenly developed motion sickness because I was no longer attuned to moving about so fast when everything had been so relaxed. And I thought that my boobs were sore because I had put so much weight back on since coming out of the jungle. Looking back on it now, it is amazing I did not realise I was pregnant, but actually the idea of it was the furthest thing from my mind.

I was more concerned about whether Gray and I would last the course.

What's happening to your body – Week 5

You: As the level of hCG being produced by your embryo begins doubling every day, pregnancy symptoms will kick in now and it is already time for you to start looking after yourself and getting lots of extra sleep.

Your baby: By the end of this week the embryo in your tummy – which is now one structure that looks a bit like a tadpole and measures about the same size as a grain of rice (5mm) – already has a beating heart, kidneys, a liver and even little buds which will form its arms and legs.

Week 6

The Week I Discovered I Wasn't Mad – I Was Pregnant

We had been fighting all evening and were exhausted. We both knew that what we really needed was a heart-to-heart but, instead, all we seemed capable of was tearing each other apart. I was terrified that if I asked Gray straight out what was really wrong he would tell me something I was dreading hearing: that he didn't love me any more. I was so sad that we seemed to have lost our wonderful relationship.

It was nearly 11 p.m. and I was lying slumped out on the sofa when suddenly I had what I can only describe as a cartoon 'light bulb' moment!

Feeling a little light-headed, I said to Gray, 'Go and get me a pregnancy test.'

'I'll go and get you one tomorrow,' he replied bitterly, convinced that I was just trying to get him out of the house.

'You know I can't be seen getting one, please go and get me one NOW,' I begged him.

With that, he turned on his heel and slammed the door.

While he was out, the thoughts started whizzing through my head and I just knew that I was pregnant. Things that had seemed so confusing suddenly made sense – the fact that I was so emotional, that my boobs were hurting like hell (other books may say 'a little tender' but all I know is that mine felt like they were on fire), that I felt so ill and exhausted.

This wasn't what pregnancy was like in the movies but, all the same, it was the only way to explain why I had changed so much.

I thought of every fight Gray and I had had, everything we'd put ourselves through, how we had come close to splitting up and now, at last, I had a reason why – I was pregnant.

It seemed like an age until Gray returned with the pregnancy test, which he had hidden between the pages of a magazine after spotting someone he knew.

I took it from him and went into the bathroom – but we had another argument because I wanted to do it alone and he wouldn't get out of the room. 'Fine, then,' I stormed. 'Stay there.'

So I sat on the toilet and did the test and within seconds the blue line had come up. I was stunned – I was right. I looked at Gray, who was sitting in the doorway, and I had a hot flush.

'Well?' he said. I asked him to give me two minutes and he folded his arms and refused, saying, 'No, I'm part of this too.'

'You're going to be a daddy,' I told him as the tears welled up in my eyes.

We were both gobsmacked. Gray slumped to the floor looking dazed and then jumped up, shouted, 'Yes, yes, yes!' and gave me a big hug, the best one we had had for weeks. Just to make sure it was no mistake, we did another test.

We then talked and talked and talked. We sat on the sofa with the lights off and the two positive pregnancy tests in front of us and we discussed everything that had happened. We backtracked on all the arguments we'd had. We talked rationally to one another for the first time in weeks and we apologised to each other for everything we had said.

My tip We started spreading our news before we even had time to take things in ourselves. My advice would be to savour your little secret between the two of you for at least a day. Give yourself time to get used to the idea of being parents – and enjoy the new feeling of becoming a family of three. And while many people like to tell their close family their good news straightaway, others may prefer to wait until the relative safety zone of the second trimester.

Gray was so ecstatic that he was jumping around but I was in total shock. I thought I was a woman who knew her own body, only to discover I didn't even know my own brain.

But we were both so relieved because we had pushed each other so far – it wasn't us, it was my hormones.

We were in a dreamlike state and immediately decided that we had to tell my parents, straightaway. By now it was past midnight but we drove across London from our flat on the Thames to my parents' house in north London. Gray was going at about twenty miles an hour – we were both aware that it was no longer just the two of us but also our baby inside me.

When we got to my parents we told them to keep September free as we might be needing a baby-sitter. Convinced that we had come round to tell them we had finally set a date for our wedding they looked at us like they didn't understand.

'We're having a baby, I'm pregnant,' I beamed at them. The only thing my shocked father could say in response was: 'My word.'

The celebrations went on until 4 a.m. – with my brother Don

and sister Jessie both arriving at the house to join in – and then we rang Gray's family in Ireland.

Everyone was so happy. Not only because we were having a child, but also because they knew how badly we had been getting on.

We had gone to the max. At least we knew why we had been fighting – although, as we were to discover, that was far from the end of the tears.

What's happening to your body – Week 6

You: The hormonal changes continue apace and you may find yourself being more emotional than ever before. You will also be exhausted as your body is working hard to sustain your pregnancy, with your heart pumping as much as 50 per cent more blood volume into your arteries. This increased blood flow passes through other organs such as the kidneys, causing you to need the toilet more often. Nausea may be making you feel a bit low. Try to get plenty of rest and eat well – even if you are suffering from morning sickness.

Your baby: Is now between 5 and 10mm – about the size of a lentil – and is beginning to look more human, although its head is as big as the rest of its body. There are dark spots where the eyes, nose and ears will be while its hands and feet look like little paddles. Halfway through this week it will make its first movements.

January 2007
Gray's Diary

This was the day it all happened. We were going through a bad patch, fighting over nothing and not enjoying being around each other. Sitting on the sofa when Leenie tells me to go and get her a pregnancy test. I say to wait until morning but she wants it now. Off I go to Tesco to buy two kits. Get them; they are in two big perspex boxes with security tags to stop people nicking them. This is a problem for me — I wanted to buy them at the self-service and not go to the checkout in case people see me buying them. Most people in here know I'm with Leenie. So I queue up and a bloke behind me goes, 'Alright Gray.' I'm gutted — it's a mate from the gym. I say hello, trying to hide these great big boxes. I'm busted — he looks at them, then we start talking rubbish — anything to stay away from the subject.

Get to the front and a woman scans the boxes but the security tags won't open for her. She rings a bell and down comes the manager to help. I want the ground to swallow me up — I knew this was a bad idea. Finally get them out of the shop. Hand them straight to Leenie and she goes to the toilet. I wait by the door. I don't believe she's pregnant but I hope to God she is. I have to play it cool just in case she isn't (or she is and doesn't want to be).

Then I push open the door. 'What's the verdict?' I ask. 'Get out,' she says. I won't move so she does it and then she says, 'You're gonna be a dad.' I sit on the floor in shock for a second or two then scream out loud, 'Yes, yes, yes!' I can't believe it's happening.

Week 7

The Week I Realised I Had Done Everything Wrong

I had about one blissful day of happiness about my pregnancy before panic set in. Although I have lots of friends who have been pregnant and always thought I'd been involved by buying them babygrows and doing baby-sitting, I suddenly realised how little I knew about what being pregnant meant.

I decided to take action after putting some body lotion on before, almost by accident, reading the back and seeing the label: 'Do not use if pregnant'. I quickly showered it off but was terrified that the damage might already be done.

The first thing I needed to do, I decided, was buy a book.

But even that was problematic. As soon as I went into Mothercare and started looking at the book section someone came up to me and asked: 'Ooooh, is it for you?' I stuttered that it was for a friend and ran out feeling mortified. I realised that if I was spotted buying a book about pregnancy the news could be leaked before I even had time to get used to the idea.

I came home to Gray really upset. 'I can't even go and get a book, no one understands,' I told him. He took the hint and went out and bought me one.

But as I started reading it, my head started throbbing, my mouth went dry and the tears welled up yet again. Everything in the book was 'Don't do this, don't do that.' I realised that I had done everything WRONG.

Terror number one was that I had pickled my baby. The night after I came out of the jungle – hours after we conceived – we had been out drinking with the winner Matt Willis and his girlfriend Emma Griffiths until the early hours.

And even more recently, I had drunk myself sober on New Year's Eve. I was so miserable about my rows with Gray that my cousin and I had been up drinking until 7 a.m.

But that was far from all. I had climbed up ladders, eaten pâté, massaged essential oils on myself, taken saunas and hot baths, been near mammals when they had given birth (the joys of television presenting) and had not taken any folic acid.

Just a couple of weeks before I found out I was pregnant I had been ill with an awful cold and I had taken every remedy under the sun – almost all of them were blacklisted by the book.

I felt rubbish. I wondered how everyone else managed pregnancy. I realised that all my friends who had children knew so much more than me – and I couldn't even ask their advice as we wanted to keep things secret.

Before I was pregnant I didn't even know what a trimester was – I'd heard the phrase vaguely bandied about before. There was so much more to being pregnant than I had ever imagined – it was a totally untapped world – and I thought that forty weeks wasn't long enough to educate myself.

I asked Gray to get me more books and magazines. But they only made things worse. The books were either too technical or too fluffy.

None of them seemed to give me the answers I needed and none described how I was really feeling. I had hoped they would give me some consolation – instead they made me feel more

My tip *If you are anything like me you are going to buy books – you've already bought this one – and it is worth your while educating yourself about the whole new world of pregnancy. You are going to worry – it is part of pregnancy. All I can suggest is that it is almost impossible to stick to all of the rules all of the time. And remember that a lot of the rules err on the side of caution – simply because no one knows what effects certain things can have on an unborn baby. It is your baby and your body and I do think that at a certain level you have to go with your gut – you know what is best for your baby, better than anyone else.*

isolated and worried. It was almost like they were tapping into my fears and distorting them. My powers of reason totally went out of the window.

Even worse, there was conflicting advice in the books and I was totally confused.

One thing I wanted to know about was exercise as, after coming out of the jungle, I wanted to stay fit. Most said do gentle exercise, but what did that mean? I presumed I couldn't go running, as you wouldn't run with a baby, but then I remembered seeing a woman in a marathon with a picture of a scan on her T-shirt saying 'Baby on board'.

A lot said to use your discretion but I could only think, 'What discretion?' I was so confused that I barely knew what day it was.

Even something you think would be simple like getting folic acid was problematic. When I went to the chemist there were millions of different pills. I was confused about whether I needed extra iron or not, about whether I needed omega-3, about what supplements to get.

I'm not much of a worrier but now I felt like I'd had a personality transplant – I could not stop panicking about my unborn baby.

I know this is not uncommon – and often it is not without reason. Lots of my friends have had miscarriages and I also know plenty of people whose babies have been born ill. What's more, my own brother was born very prematurely – my father had to deliver him at home two and a half months early.

Being pregnant was so incredible and I wanted to do everything right, so I was heartbroken to discover how difficult it was.

What's happening to your body – Week 7

You: Even the most eagle-eyed friend may not be able to notice the change in you but by now your breasts will have grown and your nipples turned darker. Once you feel you have started to grow out of your bras you will need to go and get measured for maternity ones. You will probably have to make several of these trips during pregnancy. Obviously your boobs are not the only area of growth: you may have already had to say goodbye to your waist for the next eight months. As your uterus starts growing – which can lead to some period-like cramping – you are already likely to find it impossible to fit into some of your tighter clothes and will need to unbutton the top of your trousers.

Your baby: Is now about 1.25cm – the size of a grape. Its fingers and toes are starting to develop with webbing in between them, and the teeth and palate are forming. If you could take a camera into your uterus you would be able to see all your baby's veins as its skin is still paper-thin.

Obviously Gray got the brunt of all my fears. He told me I could read the books for another week and then he took them off me. He also made it very clear to me that I was setting myself up to fail if I became obsessed on doing everything right. And he tried to calm me down by reminding me that women have been having babies for centuries.

It helped me put things into perspective but, obviously, the worrying was set to continue.

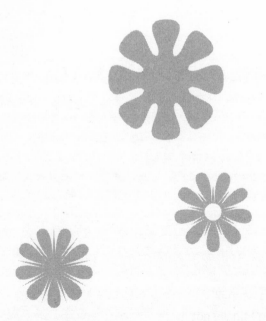

Week 8

The Week I Broke the News to My GP – and There Were More Tears

The second thing I thought I had better do now I was pregnant was go and see the doctor. I wasn't exactly sure what she would do but, as pregnancy was a medical-type-thing, I thought I had better see an expert.

My mum is a nurse so I naturally presumed that I would have my baby in our local NHS hospital and all would be hunky-dory.

Now I didn't expect my GP to roll out the red carpet for me but I hoped to have someone I could confide my fears in and who would help reassure me. Instead, my first experience was an absolute nightmare and sent me running – out of desperation – to the private sector.

Firstly I expected that she would check me. Having spoken to friends I now know that it is normal practice for your doctor simply to take your word for the fact you are pregnant, but the whole time I was sitting in the waiting room I was worrying, 'Oh God, what if I'm wrong?'

So when I finally got in to see the doctor and announced I was pregnant I expected her to do something. Instead she refused as she was 'too busy' and there was 'no need'; she asked me when it was due. How was I supposed to know?

When I said I guessed sometime in September she gave an exasperated sigh and asked, 'Well, when was the date of your last period?'

Feeling increasingly flummoxed and with tears beginning to prickle at the edge of my eyes, I looked at Gray to see if he could tell me what date I had flown home from the jungle so I could work out the exact day.

'What are you looking at him for?' she barked at me. 'You're supposed to know.' I couldn't believe how horrible she was being.

Matters went from bad to worse when I asked if correspondence to me could be sent to my house under a different name because for months somebody had been breaking into my post. I even offered to provide the envelopes.

She refused point-blank and she also made it clear that there would be no leeway around scans – I had to have them when I was told to go, which would have been impossible with my work schedule.

By now I had more or less determined that I would not be having my baby with this GP and asked her for a referral letter in case I wanted to go to a private hospital.

'You can come back and get it in two days,' she snapped.

I couldn't understand why she was being so mean and even Gray was furious at the way she was talking to me. As the tears I had been holding back popped out of my eyes she practically threw a box of tissues at me and glared.

Gray grabbed me and said, 'Come on, we're going.' I have been too embarrassed to go back to the surgery since.

By then we had decided to tell my manager that I was pregnant. It was impossible not to, as my work diary was already getting full around my due date. Jonathan was an absolute angel – could not

My tip Your pregnancy is the most incredible experience you will probably ever have and you need to have someone who understands that. Most of my friends have had good experiences in the NHS and I was just unfortunate that perhaps my GP was having a bad day – maybe she was pregnant! I was lucky to be able to move to the private sector but everyone does have choices. If you don't like your GP you can ask to see another one and there are now more choices than ever about where you can have your baby: in a hospital, a low-risk birth unit or even at home.

have been more happy – and he introduced us to our obstetrician Peter Mason.

The first time I saw him was a totally different experience from my meeting with the GP.

'Well done you,' he said when I walked into the room. I felt so proud.

He helped us choose the Lindo Wing, which is the private part of St Mary's Hospital. I was keen to choose a hospital with NHS special care because of what had happened with my brother, who had ended up being in an incubator for weeks.

There was no problem putting my details under an assumed name (which was normally Angela Quinn, as Angela is my middle name and Quinn is Gray's surname) and I could have my scans when I wanted them.

The first time I saw Dr Mason he did an internal exam and urine test to confirm that I was pregnant. I had written a whole list of the things I had done wrong and he helped calm me down.

He explained not to worry about the sauna and hot baths – that I was not about to boil the baby but the important thing was to not get too hot myself as this could lead to me becoming dizzy. He also told me about how, when it comes to medication and cosmetics, so many things are just not known, asking: 'Are you going to find fifteen hundred pregnant women to test this product on?' He said I should stop worrying so much as it was highly unlikely I had harmed my baby.

And he also set my mind at rest about my drinking – reassuring me that it was very common for women to drink before they know they are pregnant.

I had an embarrassing moment with him on my second visit when, after the thorough examination previously, I presumed I would be getting that every time. When he led me onto the same couch and asked me to 'make myself comfortable' before closing the curtain around me I immediately assumed he meant to strip off again. I was wearing a long maxi-dress so I just took it off.

As I lay there naked apart from a bra, he poked and prodded my tummy for about thirty seconds, said 'Aha', and then he was done. I was mortified, although Gray thought it was hysterical.

But even though being with Dr Mason was amazing, there were still – obviously – emotional moments.

When I had to fill the form in for the Lindo I had to put my status as single. It felt horrible and I could feel another round of tears about to come on. I sat on the sofa, turned to Gray and said, 'See, this is why we need to be married now,' and he said, 'That's not a reason to get married.'

He was right and I know we will get there in the end but I felt a real stigma attached to having to put 'single' and it seemed so cold, because it was like Gray had been written out of the equation.

However, shortly after filling out the form something happened which made us feel closer together than ever before – we saw our baby for the first time.

Dr Mason suggested we had a scan so we would know exactly how pregnant I was. Gray and I were so new to this pregnancy business that we were hoping to see a baby. Instead we saw a tiny rice-shaped cell – it was like something out of *Finding Nemo*. But there, flashing away, was our baby's heartbeat.

The doctor doing the scan said she had not seen one so clearly before – and we left her office bursting with pride and excitement. From this moment on we referred to the little baby growing inside me as rice.

What's happening to your body – Week 8

You: You are probably already having lots of mood swings – feeling angry and irritable one moment and giddy with happiness the next. This is partly due to all the extra hormones your body is producing as well as the fact that the idea of your pregnancy is still sinking in. Although your hormonal behaviour will continue throughout your pregnancy, it is most pronounced in the first trimester. The extra hormones and worry can also result in vivid dreams. Meanwhile, your progesterone levels will also be increasing which, among other things, will relax the muscles in the bowels and uterus, causing constipation. You should eat a diet rich in fibre and include plenty of liquid. That is the best way of guaranteeing normal intestinal activity.

Your baby: Is now officially a foetus and the tail it had as an embryo has gone. It measures about 1.6cm long – about the size of your thumbnail – and is undergoing huge changes this week. Almost all of its organs, muscles and nerves are beginning to function. Its arms now bend at the elbow and its eyelids and nose are forming.

Week 9

The Week I Covered a Market in Regurgitated Mango

It was 10 a.m. and Gray was driving me to work because I was feeling sick.

Suddenly I knew that I actually had to puke there and then – never mind that we were on a dual carriageway and there was a police car behind us.

As I went to open the door mumbling, 'I've got to puke,' I didn't even care that we were still driving at 50mph. But Gray, screaming, 'What the hell do you think you are doing?' pulled my hand away from the door and, with the car's wheels screeching, he swerved into the first place he could stop.

I didn't even look to see where I was before I pushed the car door open and puked my guts out. It was luminescent orange – the remains of the mango I'd had for breakfast.

Then the fuss started. My regurgitated food had landed inches away from a food market stall that was setting up.

Understandably, the stallholder was not very happy and was voicing his anger. Gray, meanwhile, was muttering furiously about how badly prepared I was as he searched my car frantically for water and wipes to help clear up me and the mess I had made.

The policemen who had followed us had got out of their car and were looking at me disdainfully. One made a sarcastic jibe about how I obviously could not take all the celebrity partying.

I was still puking and retching and, as I could hear people gradually recognise me and pull their mobile telephones out to take pictures, I didn't dare lift my head up. I was mortified.

I told Gray I wanted to clean up the mess but he snapped, 'You've nothing to clean it with,' and with that he apologised to everyone, slammed both doors shut and we drove off.

The morning went from bad to worse. After getting into work I just about managed to say: 'Good morning, you are listening to Classic FM, this is Myleene Klass,' before I had to throw my microphone down and go running into the toilet.

But while I was in there throwing up, the fire alarm went off and one of the station's staff was banging on the door, calling, 'Myleene, come out, you've got to come out, come out.' I could hear people whispering that maybe I was bulimic, and I was too scared to show my face.

Eventually I left the toilet and quietly grunted to my producer that I must have food poisoning.

Oh, the joys of morning sickness.

Now, I said at the start of this book that I aimed to be as honest with you as I could. So please allow me to dispel some myths about morning sickness. I apologise in advance if you find this a little depressing.

Morning sickness doesn't just happen in the morning: I would feel sick from five minutes after I woke up in the morning until I went to bed. It was so constant that if it didn't hit me after five minutes I was worried that something was wrong.

I prefer to refer to it as 'Mourning Your Old Life Sickness'. You want to lie in your bed and die. Because you feel green with nausea you are snappy and irritable. It turned me into a woman I didn't like that much.

My tip If you are one of the 85 per cent of pregnant women suffering from morning sickness I know you don't want to eat – but you must. The best way to do it is little and often. Towards the end of my pregnancy I got to the stage where I had to eat every hour. I also found it helped to constantly sip either water or orange juice instead of glugging it down. I had to always be putting something into my tummy. Everywhere I went I was laden down by biscuits, bananas and popcorn. I would also make sure that I ate proper meals. There is science behind this – when your stomach is empty it has nothing to digest but its own lining, which can trigger nausea,

You might not actually be sick. Most of the time I just felt nauseous and I don't know if that is actually worse because you are constantly waiting to be sick, hoping that it will bring some relief. However, when I did vomit I only felt better momentarily before the nausea would return.

Also, morning sickness doesn't immediately disappear as soon as you enter your second trimester. I was waiting for weeks and weeks for it to end – 'Any day now, any day now,' I was thinking as the weeks passed – and my sickness remained. I spoke to a nurse and said, 'I can't do this any more.' She told me: 'You could end up like me, I had it for seven months.' Not what I wanted to hear.

With me, just when I thought it was going to stay with me for the entire pregnancy, it disappeared overnight when I was four and a half months pregnant.

I was ecstatically happy for two months – it was like someone as can low blood sugar. It may be a cliché to suggest crackers and ginger biscuits as the best foods but they really worked for me. Other popular remedies for morning sickness include:

- Sniffing or eating lemons
- Drinking ginger tea
- Acupressure bands, which can be bought from your chemist
- Eating only what you think you can tolerate
- Smelling fresh mint
- Acupuncture, acupressure, meditation and hypnosis
- Cutting out coffee

had drawn open a blind and I finally felt well and healthy and happy. And then, as soon as I hit my third trimester, it returned like an evil stalker.

You may think that if you don't eat you will feel better – as there will be nothing to puke – but I discovered that the only way to stave off my feeling of sickness was to have something in me constantly. The only way I could get out of bed was to have a pack of crackers beside me. My favourite foods became crackers and ginger biscuits. I also found most dry carbohydrates and apples helped. I needed to eat all the time.

It led to some embarrassing situations, which clearly led people to believe I was either a bit weird or had an eating disorder.

One afternoon I was filming the show *School's Out* where I had to go to my old school and talk about my time there. I was happily sitting at my old desk when I got a hot flush, even though it was a cold winter's day. I started feeling really sick and was sweating profusely.

I could hear someone grumbling about the sweat on my top lip. A make-up person came over to dab me down and all I could croak out was, 'I need a biscuit.'

A poor runner was dispatched to try and find me a biscuit while I could feel everyone looking at me bizarrely.

I bumped into one of the cameramen a few months later and he said, 'It all makes sense now but we all thought you were a little odd. You didn't ask for water but for biscuits.'

When I was doing *The People's Quiz* on BBC1 I would have Maltesers, grapes and popcorn all over my desk while everyone else would have a simple cup of tea. The director would shout down my earpiece, 'Can we put the wrappers away please, Myleene?' My fellow quiz panellist Kate Garraway told me she had never seen anyone eat so much.

One driver even complained about how much I had eaten in his car and asked my bosses at CNN to reimburse him for all the popcorn I'd munched.

I knew people were talking about how much I was eating and how I was being sick. It was becoming harder and harder to keep things a secret.

What's happening to your body – Week 9

You: Your cheeks may be rosier, due to the dilation of small blood vessels, which also means you will feel a lot hotter than you did before. A decrease in your blood pressure can leave you feeling light-headed after sudden movements and, though you may not have noticed it, you are breathing much deeper.

Your baby: Is now approximately 2.3cm long from head to bottom – about the size of a piece of penne pasta – and is almost looking like a baby. Wrists have developed, its genitals have formed and even the ears are working.

1 February 2007
Gray's Diary

Still alive. Just. This is hard work. It's weird to see the girl you know so well and love change in front of your eyes. It's like a different person has come into your life. Body-wise she looks the same. Boobs are a little bigger but that's cool. But the rest, well, where do I start? I'm slowly learning to shut my mouth and not fight back. For me this is hard, because I always answer back and will always fight my corner, but now I know I will not win. I'm trying my best to walk away and not fight, so I walk into the other room and calm down or go on runs to clear my head. I think Leenie could stab me, no problem. So for the next few months I'm hiding the knives. I will tell her I don't want her to cut her fingers and it's a safety thing for the baby.

She will agree to this and that means I will get to sleep a little easier — knowing that Psycho will not be standing over me, wanting my blood.

Week 10

The Week I Panicked
at the Airport

So there I was standing in front of the airport X-ray machine, a place I had been hundreds of times before, feeling nothing less than absolute panic.

I was nauseous, I was exhausted and my head was still swimming with everything that had been happening over the last few weeks.

And I had suddenly thought that maybe there was some rule about pregnant women not being allowed to walk through the airport metal detector. I was so confused about what I could and couldn't do that I wondered whether they had a special system for women who were expecting.

I knew there was something about pregnant women and X-ray machines – just a few days earlier I had to make up a ridiculous excuse to get out of having one at the dentist. And the more I thought about it, I couldn't remember whether I had ever seen a pregnant woman walk through the metal detector.

As I reached the front of the queue I stopped dead in my tracks and ushered the people behind me through. I can't imagine what they were thinking. The security men were already eyeing me suspiciously but I couldn't ask them because I didn't want my secret out.

I pulled out my BlackBerry to see if I could get the answer on the internet but, as tears welled up in my eyes and I felt myself going bright red, I couldn't get it to work. I tried texting one of those 'information companies' who promise to answer any question you ask them – but after waiting for a couple of minutes for their reply it simply said: 'All medical questions should be referred to your doctor.'

By now I was becoming increasingly anxious as I thought about all the metal detectors I had unwittingly walked through in the first weeks of my pregnancy. But I was also totally panicked about missing my plane, which was for my first M&S modelling assignment in Cape Town.

I knew I was probably being silly but there was something in my brain saying, 'What if there is something that will harm the baby?' I telephoned my sister and begged her to go on the internet and look it up. She came back to me quickly and said she couldn't find anything to say it would be a risk just as – Sod's law – I saw a woman who was about five months pregnant walk through the machine looking as if she did not have a care in the world.

But that was not the end of my travelling woes.

On the plane I was surreptitiously reading a pregnancy book behind a magazine when I had another heart-stopping moment. I read that it is recommended that you don't fly at certain times in your pregnancy. I didn't remember seeing this in the other pregnancy books but I couldn't believe I was reading this WHILE I WAS ON A PLANE.

Already during my pregnancy I had flown back from Australia and had been to Paris, Val d'Isere, New York, Romania and Manchester and now I was going all the way to South Africa.

Trying to not let the panic seep through into my voice, I started questioning one of the air hostesses about whether she had a

My tip For the record (although I must remind you that I am not a doctor and if you have any worries you should consult yours) there is a slight increased risk of miscarriage if you are flying hundreds of times of year, due to more exposure to natural radiation. But, I repeat, only if you are flying HUNDREDS of times a year. Most airlines also do not like you to fly after 28 weeks of pregnancy just in case you end up delivering early. If you are planning to travel around the 28-week mark you can get a 'fit to fly' letter from your doctor or midwife. I would also advise wearing special flight socks when you do fly to keep your circulation flowing and to avoid swollen veins, which are more likely in pregnancy. You can get them in many chemists.

family and had she flown while pregnant. I felt sick as she jauntily told me, 'Oh no, they don't like us to fly when we are pregnant. It's something to do with the air pressure.'

When we landed I phoned Gray. He was furious and told me I had to stop reading any of the books and said he had seen millions of pregnant women flying. But I was nervous about it until my next checkup when I asked my doctor and he assured me that I wouldn't have harmed Rice. We continued to fly throughout my pregnancy – even when I was eight and a half months pregnant to Venice for another M&S shoot.

I have, however, found that flying with a bump isn't always easy. There's the ever-present weak bladder problem. I'm always torn between getting an aisle seat, which gives me easy access to the toilet but makes me feel a bit sick, and sitting by the window. I normally opted for a window seat – but there have been several times when I have woken up my neighbours by climbing over them.

And it seems I'm not the only confused one about what effect all that machinery might have on an unborn child.

When I have walked through the security gate most of the guards have been happy to scan their metal detector around me, but some are more cautious – choosing to prod my bump rather uncomfortably instead. The first time this happened goes down as my worst travelling story ever and – as usual – led to plenty of tears.

I had to go to the Bahamas for an M&S shoot when I was nearly five months pregnant. All went well until I reached Miami when I had a problem at customs. It appeared I had filled out the wrong form and they clearly didn't believe that this sick-looking, puffy-faced pregnant woman in front of them was the model she claimed to be. It seemed like an age until I convinced them that I was genuine – and then I got to security.

There was a mean-faced woman who clearly could not wait to get stuck into my bump, prodding and poking it in such a way that I was quite upset – but as this was America I thought I had better keep my mouth shut.

I finally got to the plane and sat down. The guy sitting next to me started talking and it became apparent that he thought we were going to Cuba. I couldn't believe that after the thorough search of my bump they had somehow allowed onto an American Airlines flight a bloke with the wrong boarding pass.

After we made the air steward aware of the error, it took three hours until the plane finally took off. By the time we got into the air I knew I would have missed my connecting flight to the small island where the shoot was taking place. But it was more than I could bear when we touched down in the Bahamas and I discovered my luggage had been lost.

I rang Gray in floods of tears (can you spot a pattern here?). He told me I had to calm down for Rice's sake. But things were about to get even worse.

The airline agreed to put me in a budget hotel that was so big guests had to wear colour-coded wristbands. After walking for what seemed like miles, I was too tired to even give a sob when I reached my room. It had clearly not been cleaned and the toilet was blocked. I was so exhausted I couldn't face trying to move rooms so fell asleep there and then on the side of the bed which had not been slept in.

I got some weird looks when I finally reached the small island where the shoot was taking place – while everyone was tanned and happy in their shorts I was miserable and exhausted and wearing a velour tracksuit and Timberland boots.

But M&S made me feel looked after and provided all the clothes I could ever need. It was also a special time because it was the first swim in the sea together for me and my baby.

What's happening to your body – Week 10

You: Your uterus has now grown from the size of an apple to that of a grapefruit and you may even be able to feel it above your pubic bone. You may feel more confident about your pregnancy as the chance of miscarriage is now down to 2 or 3 per cent – although fears about the health of your baby are likely to continue until you have a safe delivery.

Your baby: Is now a very busy bee, punching its arms and kicking its legs. It measures 3.3cm – about the size of a pen top – half of which is its oversized head. Over the next few weeks the limbs will start growing so that the body becomes more in proportion with the head.

Week 11

The Week I Snapped at Angus Deayton

Mother Nature can sometimes be a wicked old lady. Because when you're suffering from morning sickness and chronic exhaustion all you want to do is curl up in your bed.

But you can't because the first trimester is also the time when you're not supposed to tell people you are pregnant.

Gray and I were determined to keep our secret as quiet as possible for at least the first three months – and had told only our close families and my manager. But with my nausea, exhaustion, and hormonal stroppiness all at play, I know there were plenty of people I worked with during that time who must have thought I had become a complete diva.

One toe-curling example was when I appeared as a contestant on the quiz show *Would I Lie To You?* hosted by Angus Deayton. On the BBC1 show there are two teams – each with a leader – and you have to work out whether the other contestants have made true or false statements about themselves.

By Week 11 I had already started filling out and had worn a cardigan over my dress when I went to sit down. After a couple of hours' filming I was getting hot, feeling sick and I really needed the toilet. As all you pregnant ladies know, when you need the toilet, you really need the toilet, so I asked one of the producers how much longer the filming would be. He said no longer than fifteen minutes so I crossed my legs and we carried on. After fifteen minutes had elapsed and we didn't seem to be any closer to finishing I asked again how long it would be. My heart sank when he said, 'It could be another half an hour.'

By now all I could think about was going to the toilet and sticking my head under the tap. I wanted to jump up but I was aware that if I was the only person moving everybody would notice my little bump.

While my head was spinning with what my options were I heard Angus say to me, 'Myleene, do you think this is true or false?' 'False,' I told him with a strained look on my face. 'Would you care to elaborate?' he asked – as that's what I was on the show to do, not to actually decide whether it was true or false. 'No, it's false, false, false,' I said.

'OK, Myleene has taken over as team leader,' he said sarcastically. I didn't care – I just wanted to get to that toilet.

When you are used to being a strong career woman it is hard to come to terms with the fact that pregnancy has changed you. But, as I was discovering, you have no choice but to listen to your body.

A week earlier, when I had been in Cape Town, I had really struggled during the M&S shoot. As the new girl I was keen to make an effort with the other models and was delighted when they invited me out for a drink. But by the time I had finished shooting – after working from 5 a.m. to 7 p.m. – I literally couldn't do it.

I got to my hotel room and collapsed. Lizzie Jagger and Erin O'Connor were both phoning me, saying, 'Just come for one, you've got to come down,' but I couldn't move.

The next day I felt even more embarrassed. For one of the shots

> *My tip* This secret is the hardest one to keep. Really you want to shout it out and excuse everything – your behaviour, your weight gain, your constant need to go to the toilet – by shouting out 'I'm pregnant'. Some people decide they cannot keep it quiet and I applaud them. But like many other people, we were terrified that something might go wrong and were determined to at least find out that Rice was healthy and well before announcing it.

Lizzie and I had to push a tandem bike up a hill. It was hot and the bike was heavy and there came a point when I actually fell to my knees because I felt so dizzy and sick.

One of the people on the shoot came running over to check me and screamed out, 'She's hot!' like I was a delicate little flower. I was certainly wilting with shame.

I had a similar problem when I covered Paris fashion week for GMTV a few weeks later. As everything was done in such a rush there was no time to check our luggage in and we had to drag our suitcases around the shows with us.

No one helped me. As they said, 'You're a strong old girl, we saw you carrying trees in the jungle.' Meanwhile I was struggling to even carry myself up the stairs.

To compound matters, I was worried about hairspray. I was sure I had read somewhere that pregnant women should not be near hairspray – backstage at Paris fashion week, every other person was carrying a can, which I feared was poisoning my unborn baby.

And to add to my distress, this being fashion week there was – of course – no food to be had.

I managed to just about get through the day but that night, as so many other times, poor old Gray was the one who really suffered. The initial euphoria of my pregnancy had long since evaporated and although our rows were not as bitter as they were before we realised I was expecting, they got pretty heated. The pressure of covering up my symptoms was so stressful and when I got home after another exhausting day I needed to be looked after and cuddled.

As well as the sickness, I really suffered from the exhaustion in my first trimester. I would try and catnap in my dressing room or trailer but it was never enough. I would often come home and go straight to sleep – sometimes waking just to have dinner.

I felt like I had been plugged into the national grid as all the energy had been drained out of me. Sometimes I would feel too tired to even turn over in bed.

I'd tell Gray, 'I can't do this any longer.' But he was hard at work too, getting our flat ready for the baby by creating a nursery in our mezzanine level.

Living with the stress of keeping things a secret was telling on both of us. One evening we had an argument over who was going to put the bins out. Gray mistakenly dropped the bin bag on my foot – I was so furious that I threw it back at him – and it exploded midair, covering him in all our days-old food and rubbish. He walked out of the flat, slamming the door behind him.

I felt terrible for the way I was behaving towards Gray – I knew I was being a psycho – but I couldn't help it. I had no control over what was going on with my head.

It was a relief that there were a few people I worked with who knew. My hairdresser Donald could tell I was pregnant the instant he saw me. 'Honey, your hair's so dry, your boobs are bigger and your face is puffier – when's it due?' he asked.

I didn't even try and cover it up, as it was good to be able to talk things through with him. I was also worried about him colouring my hair so I could at least ask him properly about the fumes and dye. Hair colouring is one of those subjects on which the books seem to contradict each other – and it seems like the jury is out about whether it can really hurt your baby.

To play it safe, Donald diluted the solution down and kept it away from my roots.

We also told M&S quite early on as it was obvious that I wasn't going to be the skinny jungle girl they had hired for much longer. I was worried about how they would take it, but they were wonderful and said they were happy because 90 per cent of their customers were mothers.

What's happening to your body – Week 11

You: Will need to make an initial appointment for next week with your local doctor or hospital. This is known as booking in (in many hospitals this is at the same time as your first ultrasound). You also need to start thinking about what tests – if any – you may want. A dark vertical line called the linea nigra may start to develop on your stomach – it will gradually disappear once your baby is born.

Your baby: Is developing at a rapid rate and will double in size – from 4cm (the length of an AA battery) to 8cm – over the next three weeks. Minute details like fingernails and toothbuds are developing, while the fingers and toes are no longer webbed. The baby is waking and sleeping in short five- to ten-minute cycles and can already be awoken by a cough from you.

And I couldn't keep the secret from my best friend Lauren Laverne, who I first worked with on *CD:UK*. To my amazement and joy, when I announced my news to her she told me she was also pregnant – just five weeks later than me – and it has been incredible for us going through this journey together.

Gray and I were terrified the news that I was pregnant would leak before I'd had my scan, so we impressed heavily on those people who did know how important it was to keep it a secret. But this caused added stress as when our families phoned me they never asked me about the pregnancy because they never knew who could overhear. I got really upset because I thought they didn't care about it.

The only person I could openly discuss the pregnancy with was Gray. But often we were barely talking to each other.

12 February 2007
Gray's Diary

Started work on baby's room. Leenie is working most days so she is not in the way. She's so tired all the time. Not much I can do except make her life as easy as possible. But, trust me, that's easier said than done. Make her breakfast, then she tells me I use too much milk. Give her orange juice, she tells me I should use a smaller glass. I think it's my fault that the sun's not shining today. Bite my lip, help her get ready, say goodbye. Off she goes. 'Bye, bye, love ya,' I say quickly. Close the door in case she tries coming back. The poor driver has to take her to work. Feel sorry for ya, mate, but glad it's not me. Peace for me for the day, can get on with all the work. But I must not forget to text her at least twenty times during the day so she won't start a fight with me for not checking she's OK.

These months have been the hardest I have had since I was first with Leenie. She has turned into a witch. I think she could actually take flight now and turn me into a frog with one of her spells. What has happened to my girl? Where has she gone? Everything I do or say is wrong and I'm no help at all to her — so she tells me every day.

I get more friendliness from the checkout staff at the local supermarket than I do from her. I hope she really is pregnant and that all this is not for nothing because all I have seen in the last three months is her eating much more, sleeping much more and nagging everyone. I hope the next six months are not like this or I will have to take a security job in Iraq — I think I will be safer there than at home with my witch.

Week 12

The Week Rice Became Real

I woke up with my heart racing and my palms sweating. I'd been having a nightmare that I had left the baby somewhere and I could not find it. Gray was ringing on the doorbell telling me to hurry up, while I was frantically trying to remember what I had done with Rice.

Clearly I was a little anxious about our scan.

Although my pregnancy symptoms were continuing in earnest and I felt sure Rice was alive and well, scans are always a bit scary as well as being the most wonderful of things.

This time – after our last scan only showed a heartbeat – we did not know what to expect. As the doctor put the gel on my tummy we held hands in anticipation.

At first all this grey matter came onto the screen and it was hard to make head or tail of it. But as the doctor moved her stick around we could see a hand and then a leg and a foot and it was one of the most incredible experiences of my life.

Last time we had seen our baby it had been a heartbeat. Now it really looked like a little human being. I was sobbing my heart out and even hardman Gray had a tear in his eye.

One of the best things was seeing Gray's reaction. He could see that I hadn't made it all up – that I hadn't simply got a bit rounder – there actually was a baby in my tummy. Our baby.

As the doctor started measuring things like the baby's head I

My tip If you can, get your partner to come to all of your scans. It is so much harder for them to envisage what is going on inside you and the scan can change that. I found that seeing Rice properly for the first time really made Gray think about being a dad – and meant he was a bit more forgiving of my hormonal moodiness.

drove her mad with questions: 'Is that OK? Is this OK? Does that look normal?' She was – quite rightly – busy looking at the brain and the umbilical cord while I was desperate to see things like the legs and the face.

I even asked for a close-up of the leg – I loved that the baby could stretch its legs out. At one point it clenched its fists and looked like it was having a boxing match. It then turned to the camera and we saw its face. We were giggling with excitement – our baby already had a mind of its own.

Doctors don't tend to get over excited at scans – while you want your baby to be remarkable or brilliant they are happiest when everything is normal and average. Thankfully, everything was.

After our appointment we sat in Gray's car outside the hospital scouring the scan pictures, looking at our baby's arms and legs, before sending them over to both our families.

I'm not surprised some people think those twelve-week photos look more like aliens than humans but all we could see was our baby. We could see how tiny and vulnerable it was – and that it already had a personality.

I couldn't concentrate on anything else the rest of the day – all

I could think about was little Rice boxing and wiggling about in my tummy.

The scan made us both feel different. I think it was when it really hit us that we were going to be parents. From that time on both of us became a lot more careful about the dangers in our day-to-day lives – crossing roads, driving cars, getting on planes – as we knew Rice needed both its mummy and daddy.

It was also the time when I realised there was a whole world out there that I had not known existed. Suddenly, everywhere I looked, there were pregnant women or mummies with prams or

What's happening to your body– Week 12

You: Will probably get to see your baby this week at an ultrasound scan. The scan will give doctors the best estimate of how old your baby is, whether you're expecting twins (or more!), the position of the placenta and the size of the nuchal translucency. This is the measurement of the soft-tissue thickness on the back of the baby's neck. If it is thicker than average this could mean the baby has a higher risk of an abnormality such as Down's syndrome and you may be advised to have further tests to investigate. You will also have your booking-in appointment (although in some hospitals this is done at a different time) where your midwife will ask you about your medical history and lifestyle and give you blood tests to check your blood group, your iron levels, your immunity to rubella (German measles), and whether you have syphilis or hepatitis B. Your urine is also tested for bacteria.

Your baby: Now measures 5.6cm – about the size of a matchbox. Its face is beginning to look more human, with its eyes – which started at the side of the head – moving closer together towards the front. Its reflexes are beginning to work, with fingers opening and closing, toes curling and mouth sucking.

daddies with papooses. Every other advert was for nappies or for toys.

We were both so excited we were going to be part of this world. We couldn't stop talking about our baby: what its personality was going to be like, who it was going to look like.

Because it had been so boisterous at the scan Gray was convinced it was a boy.

I wasn't so sure – I had a feeling we were having a girl.

3 March 2007

Gray's Diary

Today was the best so far. We went for our second scan and got to see so much of Rice. We think Rice is a boy – he or she was boxing in one of the photos and resting in another one. It's mad to see our baby. Best feeling in the world. I wish the time would go quicker. Can't wait to hold Rice. We got four photos to take home with us. I'm over the moon.

Week 13

The Week People Started Hinting I Was Getting Fat

Although we now knew the pregnancy was progressing well, we decided to try and keep our news secret for a few more weeks. Gray wanted to fly over to Ireland to tell his friends in person while I – whose every move is well documented – wanted to keep our secret between us for just a little bit longer. I was also a little bit worried that being perceived as the 'pregnant girl' could make some people limit the sort of work I was doing. I wanted to keep going.

In retrospect, maybe we should have just announced it there and then, as the secrecy added so much to the pressure. One of the most difficult things was the struggle to keep on making excuses for my changing shape.

The poor stylist on *The People's Quiz*, which I was doing at the time, didn't know what to make of it. Every week I was getting bigger.

I could hear her muttering to herself, 'I don't understand, these fitted last week, they promised me it was a size eight.' Then we would put on a size ten dress and by the following week that would be too small. She was obviously too polite to say, 'Stop putting on weight,' so I would give a nervous laugh and shrug my shoulders, saying, 'Sorry, I must have had too many doughnuts.'

The weight was mainly going on my boobs, my bum, my waist and my hips. While my legs and arms were the same size they had always been, my tiny waist totally disappeared and my boobs shot from a D to an E.

With CNN it was even worse. I'd had to give them my exact measurements but by the time I saw them my weight had gone up and nothing fitted. I ended up bringing my own clothes into work – wrap dresses were my total saviour.

At shoots I developed a technique of getting changed with my coat on so that no one could see my stomach. But I was convinced that any woman who saw me must surely realise I was pregnant.

At home things were equally frustrating. I'd love to meet one of those women who managed to wear their normal clothes until they were seven months gone.

I was finding this transition stage really hard. At the start of the second trimester you don't have a real bump but you no longer have your figure. You have a flabby middle and just look a bit podgy. You want to shout out, 'I'm not fat, I'm pregnant!' and you look at women with really lovely big bumps with envy.

Normally I pride myself on going to my wardrobe, putting on the first dress I fancy, and then leaving the house. But now I was trying on outfit after outfit and none of them fitted.

Jeans were a complete no-no while the tops that did fit made my cleavage so high I looked like Dolly Parton. I tried to cover my little bump and my two big mountains with heavy jumpers and skirts but I looked awful – like a bag lady.

One afternoon I came into the living room with a thick polo neck over one of the few dresses that I could still wear. Gray took one look at me and – for the first time in our relationship – he begged me to go shopping, saying that I looked like I had fallen into a skip and put on the first things I'd found in it.

My tip It's that tough time when you are too small for proper maternity gear but too big for your normal clothes. The best thing to do is buy just a few clothes in a size or two bigger than you normally are. Although some people might complain that it is a waste of money, you are likely to get use out of them on the way down too – just after you have had the baby – and you can swap with friends as well. I would also say get lots of staples like vest tops – things you can layer with. The other best items in my wardrobe from this time were my wrapover dresses, which can accommodate the changes in your waist.

And if you too are suffering from erect nipples, I can't recommend nipple daisies and a bit of toupee tape enough – you should be able to get both in big department stores.

Lauren and I hit the shops like two giggly girls let out of school early. Thankfully the smock-dress fashion was in and we could buy to our hearts' content knowing that everyone was looking pregnant – not just us.

However, as my face became puffier, my weight gain was still becoming impossible to hide. People would stop me in the street or in Starbucks and make comments like, 'You look bigger in real life.' I don't think they meant to be rude – none of these things were said maliciously – but they were quite upsetting all the same.

The few people I worked with who knew my secret were also telling me what people were saying. And because I was putting on weight but often running to the toilet to be sick the rumour mill was going into overdrive that I was developing an eating disorder – it wasn't what I needed to hear.

My weight was not the only body issue which could have given me away, though.

As well as my cleavage beginning to look like Jordan's, there was also the not-so-slight problem of my huge nipples, which were now so sensitive that they were almost always erect.

On the night of the BAFTAs I was doing the red carpet for Orange, which meant walking up and down interviewing the stars in my yellow satin dress. After hours of talking to the camera my manager turned to me and whispered, 'Be careful, your nipples are showing.'

What's happening to your body – Week 13

You: Congratulations! You've reached the end of the first trimester. Many people decide to now announce to their friends and work that they are pregnant – which often will make your life easier. Your pregnancy symptoms should gradually also start to wane. Hopefully you will get to see why the second trimester is called the 'honeymoon period' as your energy returns and your nausea subsides. However, each pregnancy is different and some people will not lose their symptoms until much later.

Your baby: Is still growing rapidly and is now about 7cm long – about the size of a peach. Its ears are now almost in the right position, its unique fingerprints have developed and its bones are hardening.

I was totally mortified – the last thing I wanted to be talking about with Jonathan was my nipples. I was wearing a bra and didn't know what else to do. 'Can we not have this discussion again,' I whimpered.

But just a few days later when I was doing *The People's Quiz* the stylist made a similar comment, saying, 'Somebody has had a quiet word and your nipples are showing.'

Thankfully she had a solution – nipple daisies. They are little flower-shaped stickers that you cover your nipples with. They became my most constant friend and I normally had at least three pairs in every handbag.

So, I had my nipple daisies, I had my smock dresses and my wrapovers. I thought I was hiding things well. And then something else came along to trip me up.

Week 14

The Week I Fell Over in Boots

I was struggling to come to terms with the new way I looked. As well as the huge boobs and hips, erect nipples and puffy face, I also had hay-dry hair and had come out in spots.

My heels were my last refuge of glamour. I knew I would have to give them up soon enough – so was determined to get as much use out of them as possible.

I had already had a few moments where I felt a little uneasy on my feet. Pregnant women are usually advised to ditch their heels at around twenty weeks because the baby has caused their centre of gravity to change and also because they can lead to back pain. But as I didn't even have a sizeable bump yet I couldn't believe that it was already time to say goodbye to my lovely shoes.

Until I fell over rather spectacularly.

Now we are not talking about a little quiet trip on a pavement stone or even a graceless tumble down the stairs. This was a rather ridiculous comedy fall in the middle of a very busy branch of Boots, bringing an entire shelf of goods clattering down with me.

I had rushed into the store to buy some deodorant on my way out to lunch with Lauren. I was scooting around trying to find the right section in the knowledge that I was late. I was also wearing my magnificent three-inch high cowboy boots along with some leggings and a smock top.

Reaching out to ask a security guard where the deodorant shelf

> *My tip* As soon as you start to feel a
> little off balance it is time to
> ditch those heels. It's hard, I know. But you can get
> some really nice flatties – honestly!

was, I obviously tipped my centre of gravity a little too far and felt myself falling. My arms flailed wildly in an attempt to grab something to stop me. But it was no good. There was this terrible clang and I ended up bottom first on the floor with – coincidentally – a whole shelf of deodorants on top of me.

It was hideous. My face turned so red it felt like it was on fire. I wanted to totally disappear.

I looked up and there was a couple all dressed up in gothic gear looking at me strangely. They asked, 'Are you Myleene?' and when I nodded weakly, they said, 'What the hell are you doing?'

While they stared the gentlemanly security guard tried to help me up. But as he grabbed my torso my feet kept on slipping from under me. In the end I had to get onto my hands and knees and pick myself up.

I was shaking but offered to help clear the mess. The security guard took one look at me and made clear in no uncertain terms that I should stay well away.

The gothic pair, meanwhile, came up and asked for autographs.

When I met Lauren the first thing she asked was, 'What the hell happened to you?' There was a huge hole in the knee of my leggings. When I told her about my fall she shook her head and said, 'Leenie, time to ditch those heels.'

That was easier said than done. I had a couple of pairs of ballerina shoes in my wardrobe but within a few weeks they no longer fitted me. None of my shoes did – I had gone up by a whole size.

I was stuck wearing ugly flip-flops for weeks on end – which wasn't great in the wettest summer for years.

M&S saved me. When I let slip to someone about my footwear problem, the next day I got two suitcases full of ballerina shoes, which I lived in. The only other footwear I could walk in was trainers – although towards the end of my pregnancy Gray had to help to tie the laces.

A couple of weeks after my incident in Boots there was one more occasion when I thought I would try and wear heels. It was the Classical BRITs – the biggest night in the classical-music calendar – and I wanted to look my best.

It did not go too well. Climbing up the stairs I was saved from tumbling down only after my manager grabbed me as I started to fall. After that Jonathan insisted on holding my arm whenever we walked together – he obviously thought I was a complete liability.

What's happening to your body – Week 14

You: Are now officially in your second trimester and may be feeling much happier and less worried than you have been. This is the time when many women really start to experience the famed pregnancy glow, with rosy cheeks, glossy hair, perfect skin and healthy, strong nails.

Your baby: Is both growing (it is now 9cm long, the size of a Weetabix) and developing at great speed. This week it starts breathing amniotic fluid – it gets its oxygen directly from you – producing urine and swallowing. It is also becoming hairy – head hair and eyebrows are starting to emerge, while a downy hair called lanugo is developing on its skin. This will usually disappear just a few weeks before birth.

After that the heels were relegated to being on show only – I wore them throughout my pregnancy on *The One Show* – but only once I was sitting down. My co-host Adrian Chiles' favourite joke was that I was the only person he knew who wore heels to sit down in. My flip-flops were within reach behind the sofa along with a punnet of strawberries, a Diet Coke and a bag of nuts.

Meanwhile I could only stare at my cupboard of gorgeous shoes in despair. I'd heard that if your feet grow in pregnancy, sometimes they do not go back to their normal size after you have had the baby.

And don't even talk to me about the weight gain.

16 March 2007

Gray's Diary

Went to see Faithless in concert. Came home to see Leenie – but she got back after me. Then it started: World War Three. I should be able to stop this but I can't. The two of us screaming at each other over nothing. I feel like shit. Leenie is being so hard on me, slamming doors, getting herself into a state. This is not good for Rice. I walk away into the spare room to try and let her calm down. It's a sad night. I'm going away in the morning and we are fighting and I'm in the spare room just to keep her calm.

Week 15

The Week I Discovered I Was Craving the Wrong Things

The subject of food and drink is something no pregnant woman can steer away from.

Everyone has an opinion on what you can and can't eat, whether you should have any alcohol or caffeine, and what foods you are craving.

The books I read are full of lists of nutritious meals you should be eating and foods which are banned – and as usual they often contradict each other.

Fish is supposed to be good, except for certain types and you should only have it twice a week. There is a whole different rule for oily fish – so you can have more tinned tuna (not classed as oily) than fresh tuna (which is classed as oily).

Loading up on calcium is recommended but while you can have some hard cheeses you have to avoid soft ones altogether.

Foods containing iron are good but liver, which also has too much vitamin A, is bad.

Some people say you can have sushi and others say you can't.

You can have mayonnaise bought in a shop but avoid it if it is home-made.

If you buy pre-packed salad you have to wash it first.

As far as I can tell, the jury is out on smoked fish, cold meat, potato salad, coleslaw and Parmesan cheese.

And then there is the whole 'eating for two' or 'eating for one plus a few extra calories' row.

And people wonder why pregnant women are stressed!

My main concern was keeping my nausea at bay, so I was eating anything that didn't make me feel like gagging. So there I was, happily chomping away on my latest craving – peanut butter – and going through a jar every three days. I thought there was nothing wrong with peanut butter until I invited Lauren to join me in a jar or two and she looked shocked and told me I was supposed to be staying away from peanuts.

Where had that rule come from? I couldn't remember reading it in any of my books. I knew to avoid shellfish and goats' cheese and all of the obvious stuff. But then again the dos and don'ts food lists had been so long that I might have just skimmed past it.

So I checked with my doctor. He gently told me that it was probably best to stay off my peanut butter. Peanuts are one of those million and one things that the people who we normally rely on to know things don't know whether or not they can affect the unborn foetus. Women who have histories of allergies are warned to avoid peanuts because they may or may not cause your baby to become allergic to peanuts.

Cue the usual dramatics and worries that I had harmed Rice in some way before I had even got to meet him or her. If the baby does end up with a peanut allergy I know I will never forgive myself. But a few weeks after Rice was born, new studies seemed to show that babies whose mothers ate peanuts during pregnancy were less likely to have nut allergies. More confusion.

There were lots of times I was to break the food rules unwittingly. As I have already described, I started my pregnancy off being terrified I had pickled the baby after a few heavy nights of vodka and pina coladas. I ate chocolate mousse without realising it contained raw eggs, a ravioli I didn't know had goats' cheese in it and I found cream cheese almost impossible to avoid.

There were a few things I made my mind up to steer clear of. As the rules on alcohol seemed to be changing by the second, I decided to abstain completely (but God, I missed it). My thinking was that I would never give a baby a glass of wine.

But then I wouldn't give them a can of Diet Coke or a large sugary doughnut either – and they were part of my staple diet.

I just couldn't go without any caffeine. Before I was pregnant I was a coffee addict and always had a Frappucino in my hand.

The minimum I would have would be four coffees and three Diet Cokes a day. I needed my Diet Coke and had decided to allow myself one can a day, but was devastated when a total stranger came up to me after we had announced my pregnancy and started having a go at me for drinking it. 'You're out of order,' she told me. 'It's full of chemicals.'

Later on, while I was on holiday in Mauritius, I was downing a glass of orange juice (which was one of my most consistent cravings) when a woman came up to me and said I was putting my baby in danger by giving it too much vitamin C. I tried to point out that your body can get rid of vitamin C but she was having none of it.

Each time I worried I spoke to the ever-calm Dr Mason and he normally reassured me that I was not doing anything wrong. He even said that my Diet Coke was fine and was so annoyed when I told him what the stranger had said that he uncharacteristically swore: 'That's bollocks.'

But I was lucky to have him as a sounding board. They say common sense rules when you are pregnant but the irony is that

My tip I'm going to be saying this a lot – but Mama knows best. Only you can decide which of the dozens of rules to follow when it comes to eating. I did not have the time, energy or inclination to try and follow the many rules about what percentage of carbs, vegetables and calcium you should be eating – I ate what my body was craving. I figured that was obviously what my body needed.

As to what you do not eat, make your decision on things like alcohol and stick to it. I chose to avoid alcohol and things that had made me ill in the past – specifically seafood. I also stayed away from the foods that everyone agreed could make you sick, like paté, uncooked meats and soft smelly cheeses.

I'm not advocating that you put on the weight like me, but the way I see it, this is the one time you are allowed to be fat. Enjoy! And try to ignore what other people say (apart from your doctor). It's your baby and your body.

Having said that, if you are anything like me, you will still be worrying.

you are so mixed up with everything going on with your body that you have no idea what is right or wrong.

Even if you did know how to look after yourself, how do you know what's right for the vulnerable little being inside your belly?

You can drive yourself mad with worry while other people – who always have an opinion to give – either think you are being too hard on yourself or too easy. One evening I was in a sushi bar with friends and they were trying to get me to eat sushi, telling me it was fine. I felt like a complete killjoy when I insisted on only having noodles.

As for the 'How much you can eat' debate – well, I just throw my hands up in the air. Most of the books I read were more like diet manuals then pregnancy journals. I even read somewhere that you should just put weight on in your seventh month. Well,

What's happening to your body – Week 15

You: If there are any concerns about your pregnancy you will be offered further tests to be done between weeks 15 and 20. The multiple marker screening test is done on a sample of your blood and estimates the likelihood of Down's syndrome by measuring the levels of alpha-fetoprotein or AFP – a protein produced by the foetus – among other things. If the likelihood of Down's syndrome or any other chromosomal abnormality is found to be high then you will be offered either an expert ultrasound assessment or amniocentesis. This involves passing a needle into the amniotic sac under ultrasound guidance to pick up loose cells from the baby which are floating in the amniotic fluid. Those cells are then tested to determine whether they have any abnormality.

Your baby: Now measures about 11cm, the size of a mobile phone, and its reproductive organs are developing. Girls will develop up to six million eggs in their ovaries during gestation but that will have gone down to one million by the time they are born. In boys the prostate gland is developing and genitals are becoming more defined. Also this week the facial muscles become active and your baby will make involuntary grimaces, squints and frowns, and may even be able to suck its thumb.

never one to do things by halves, I put on two stone by month five and more than four stone by the end of my pregnancy.

As I have already explained, I needed to eat constantly. And although one of my cravings was apples – it had to be Pink Ladies because of the crunchy taste – most were not anywhere near as healthy.

Ginger biscuits, crackers, popcorn, pizza and salty chips were all my favourite things. I could quite easily down four bowls of Frosties every day. I needed lots and lots of carbohydrates. Protein most often came in the form of spaghetti Bolognese, which I would crave at all hours of the day. And I had a baked potato, cheese and baked beans every day without fail.

Orange juice was also one of the biggies. I always had to have some orange juice near me and normally drank around one and a half litres a day.

There was no way I could keep an eye on the calories I was consuming as I was eating so much. Gray used to joke that the only thing I hadn't forgotten in my pregnancy was the way to the fridge.

I gave up caring that I was breaking the rules about how much to eat. Not feeling sick was more important to me. And then I got ambushed by the cold from hell.

Week 16
The Week I Felt Like I Was Dying

I felt like I had an elephant sitting on my chest, there were razor blades in my throat and my bones were aching.

It was nothing more than a common cold but I felt one hundred times worse than I have ever done before.

I wasn't comfortable in bed but my head was pounding so much that I couldn't bear to move. The thing I wanted to do more than anything else was totally knock myself out. But I wasn't even sure whether I was allowed to use some Vicks.

Perhaps even more problematic than the 'What you can or can't eat' debate is the 'What medicine you can have' debate. I'm not one of those people who happily pops a pill at the slightest sign of a sickness and now that I was pregnant I wanted to even less. But I was feeling so ill that I honestly felt like I was dying.

I am normally pretty healthy and I attribute that in part to the fact that I spend so much time running around there is no time to get ill. It is only when I take a break that my immune system packs up – every time I have a holiday, without fail, I get a cold.

But this time I had got stuck broadcasting in the rain and, even though I had done my best to stay as dry as I could, I knew that I would end up ill from it.

And being ill is so much worse when you're pregnant. Some

My tip If you have a cold the best thing to do is totally rest. You need to sleep more than ever as it will be so much harder to get well again. Aside from Vicks, most cold medication is out, so it is back to the old-fashioned methods to help alleviate your symptoms. You should:

- Drink lots of fluids
- Try and eat – especially things containing vitamin C
- Use extra pillows to help you breathe as you sleep
- Suck on sweets and gargle with salt water
- As well as rubbing Vicks on your chest you can also use it as a decongestant by putting it in water and inhaling
- Some people swear by nasal strips to help you breathe – you can get these in most chemists

doctors think your immune system is already low to stop your body rejecting your baby. And your baby mops up all the goodness left in you for itself – you are left with nothing.

I was still experiencing the constant nausea and exhaustion and with this terrible cold on top I felt awful.

The icing on the cake was the fact that all the medications I would normally have reached for were out of bounds.

As there have not been any tests on them, you are advised to steer clear of most of the cold medications. Every one of my old favourites, I now spotted, had the line, 'Do not use if pregnant or breastfeeding without consulting your doctor.'

If your sickness does not disappear after ten days get a checkup with a doctor. Also watch out for sinusitis, which is common in pregnant women after colds — symptoms include tenderness beneath the eyes, headaches, toothache and thick mucus.

Symptoms for urinary tract infections can often be 'silent' like mine were, but if you have any cystitis-like symptoms — a strong urge to urinate even more than normal but not really needing to go, a burning sensation when using the toilet and sharp pain in the abdominal area — make sure you go and see your doctor.

After three days of torture and Gray force-feeding me lemon tea I was contemplating putting some Vicks on. There were no warnings on it — only that it should not be given to children under six months. But I was still worried.

I felt too embarrassed to phone my doctor so Lauren volunteered to call her hospital and ask for me, as she didn't know either. The midwives laughed and said, yes, I could have Vicks.

When Lauren called me back we laughed too at how silly I was being. But, like almost everything to do with pregnancy, it was so confusing that it's not surprising that I was worried.

Much later on in my pregnancy, I got sick again — but this time I didn't even realise it. While in Venice for my M&S shoot I'd had a few stabbing pains in my tummy and I was also a lot more tired. But I put it down to being in the later stages of pregnancy (by then I was 36 weeks) and thought nothing of it.

Then when I went for my routine test at the hospital they found some protein in my urine. They didn't seem overly concerned and I carried on with work. But when I came home from doing The One Show I had a message saying I needed to get hold of some antibiotics straightaway as I had a urine infection.

I was heartbroken that having got so far in my pregnancy I was going to have to take drugs. But after speaking to Lauren and my neighbour, who is a nurse, I realised I had better do it – if left untreated urinary tract infections can lead to kidney disease and early labour.

It was a lot easier being ill the second time round as at least there were lots of people I could turn to for advice.

Although advice, as I was about to discover, could be a mixed blessing.

What's happening to your body – Week 16

You: Now that your pregnancy is safer and you are feeling more energetic it is a good time to think about some gentle exercise which may help you keep fit and enable you to cope with the pains to come – particularly back pain caused by the weight of your baby. Pregnancy yoga, walking and swimming are all good, gentle ways to keep fit without working up too much of a sweat.

Your baby: At 11.7cm your baby is the size of an avocado and weighs about 3oz. This week your baby will start hiccupping – a precursor to breathing. This will continue throughout your pregnancy and when your baby is big enough you will regularly be able to feel it. Your baby is also becoming more sensitive to light, although its eyes are still fused together.

Week 17

The Week People Questioned Whether My Pregnancy Was an April Fool Joke

It was 6.30 p.m. on a Saturday night and Gray was in Dublin breaking the news to his extended family and friends. The phone was ringing but, enjoying the chance to get stuck into my piano practice without any distractions, I ignored it.

By the time I picked it up I realised that life was not going to be the same again.

It was a female journalist from a Sunday newspaper. Although she didn't say why she had called, the message was curt but friendly: 'Hi Myleene, please could you give me a call as I need to ask you something.' I knew the secret was out.

I rang Simon Jones, my publicist, to say he needed to release the story straightaway, and then I rang Gray to say he had better tell everyone quickly as the story was going to be in the next day's papers.

It wasn't how we had planned to release the news – we were going to do it the day later in a press release as we wanted everyone to have the news at the same time – but by now we were ready.

However the fact that it ran on 1 April, April Fools' Day, led to some really strange comments. I woke up on the Sunday morning to see headlines plastered all over the newspapers about my

My tip Only you can decide when the best time to share your news is. You might want to tell all your friends straightaway or you might be ultra-cautious like we were and wait until you're nearly five months. But I do have to stress how wonderful it was to be able to have my bump out. It is also worth remembering that to qualify for statutory maternity pay you must tell your employer at least fifteen weeks before your due date. By law they must give you time off for antenatal appointments and classes. It is against the law for your boss to treat you unfairly, sack you or make you redundant because of your pregnancy.

Now is also a good time to check out your maternity pay. All employed mothers have the right to 26 weeks off called Ordinary Maternity Leave

pregnancy. The headlines ranged from 'Myleene pregnant' to my favourite, 'Ante-natal Klass'.

That afternoon I was driving with my cousin to lunch at my parents' house when we heard my name being mentioned on the radio. We turned it up and couldn't believe what we were hearing.

'I don't think Myleene is pregnant – she wouldn't do that sort of thing,' one guy was saying. Huh? I wouldn't procreate?

'Yes, it is definitely an April Fool,' said another. 'She doesn't look pregnant in any of the pictures.'

There was a whole debate about whether or not I was pregnant. My cousin and I couldn't believe it – it wasn't as if the idea of me being pregnant was really funny – or was it?

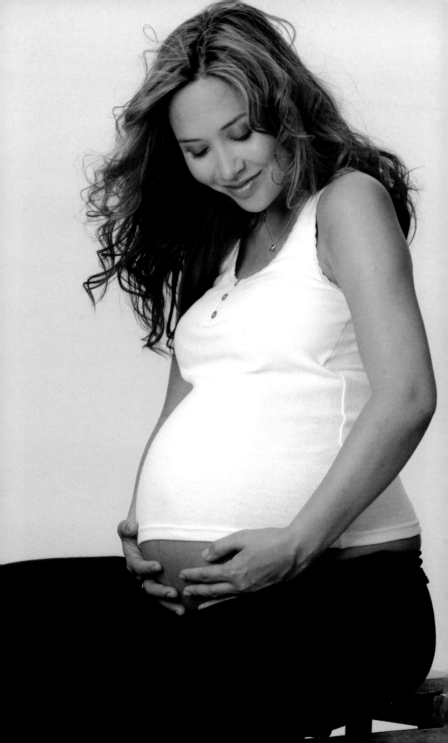

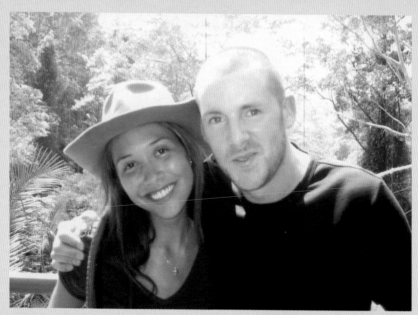

It was a brilliant surprise to see Gray when I came out of the jungle.

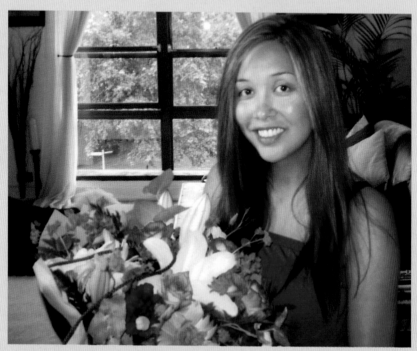

We were over the moon when we realised I was pregnant.

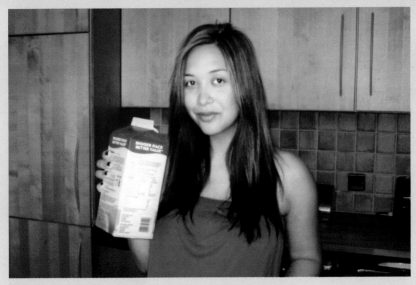

The lists of what you can and can't eat and drink are so confusing.
I drank orange juice constantly throughout my pregnancy.

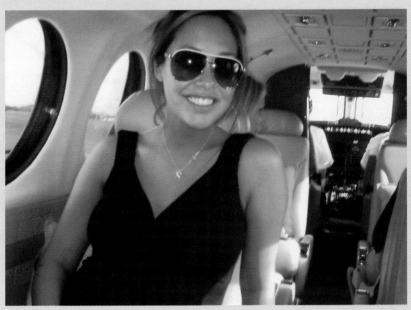

I also flew throughout my pregnancy.

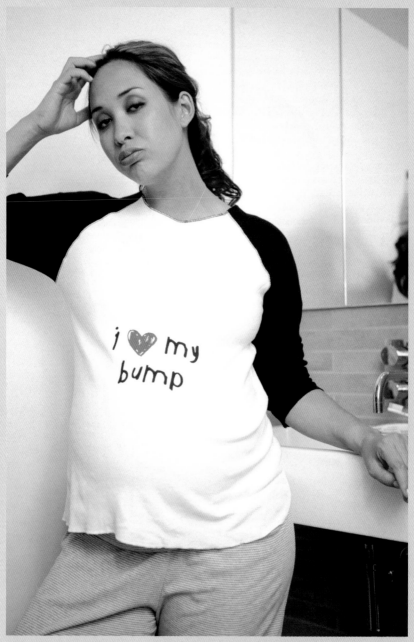

Morning sickness – which comes at any time of the day.

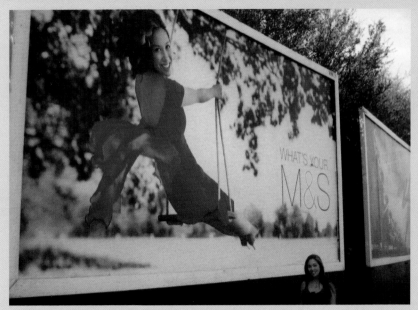

I look so peaceful on the swing but I was actually feeling really sick.

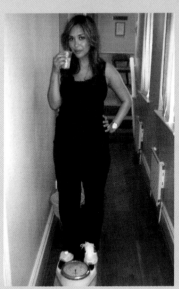

I was struggling to keep my growing bump under wraps.

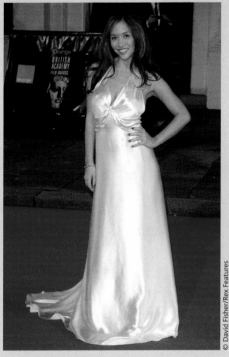

Me at the Baftas: Next time I will know to wear my nipple daisies.

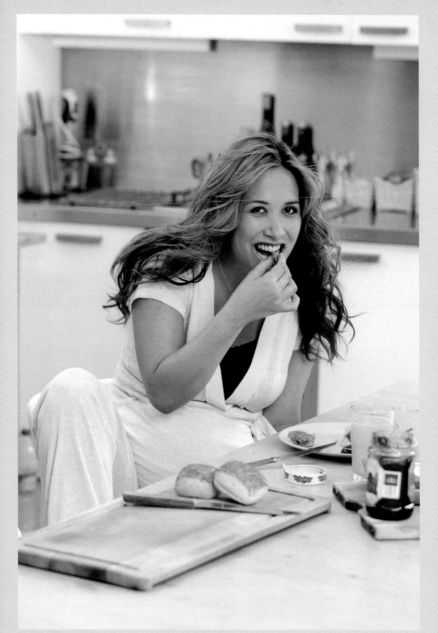

Gray joked the only thing I didn't forget while I was pregnant was my way to the fridge –
I was always eating.

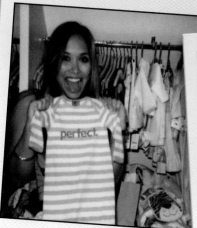

Everyone's generosity was incredible.

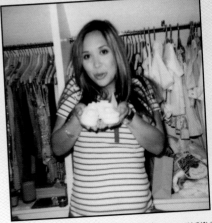

Finally an excuse to buy twice as many shoes, albeit much smaller ones.

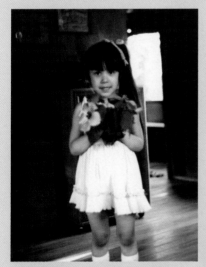

Me in the Philippines. I look like butter wouldn't melt in my mouth but I stole the one toy my cousins owned. I still remember the almighty telling off I got.

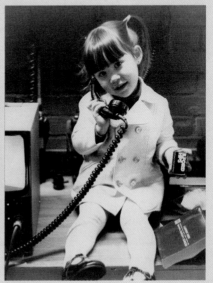

I always loved a good gossip.

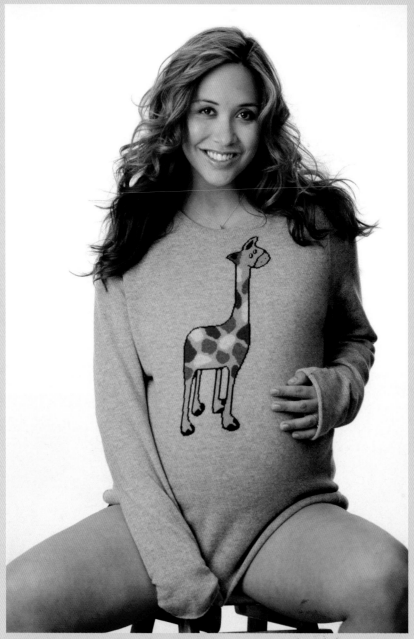

Growth spurt: I couldn't believe how big I got.

(OML), when all your employment rights are the same as if you were still at work, and a further 26 weeks called Additional Maternity Leave (AML), when your rights to things such as pension and holiday pay are no longer applied.

Statutory Maternity Pay (SMP) is available for women who have worked continuously for an employer for 26 weeks up to 15 weeks before their due date. Although you will need to read your contract to see exactly what you are entitled to, by law companies have to pay 90 per cent of your salary for the first six weeks followed by a weekly flat rate. In 2007/8 that rate was £112.75. If your earnings per week are less than the flat rate then you will receive 90 per cent of the flat rate. SMP is paid for the first 39 weeks of your leave.

That evening, when I did my own radio show for Capital FM, I decided to announce it myself to stop any more silly talk about my pregnancy being a joke.

Once the news was officially out, Gray and I were able to breathe a big sigh of relief. It was nice to know people would realise all my strange behaviour was down to the fact that I was pregnant and not a gluttonous nutter. It was like an instant weight had been taken off my shoulders and it was such a relief to be able to walk down the street with my belly out.

And when, a few days later, my nausea also began to lift, I felt like a different person altogether. I became madly in love with Gray all over again and started to actually enjoy being pregnant.

My skin cleared up, my energy levels improved, my hair became silky and I almost forgot what being sick was like. I could see why people call the second trimester the 'honeymoon period'.

But the best thing about everyone knowing was how special people made me feel, and how wonderful and supportive perfect strangers were about my pregnancy. I was also astounded, amazed and totally gobsmacked about the letters and gifts that I started receiving.

Adorable baby blankets started arriving by the truckload. I got scores of presents from well-wishers. Women of all ages wrote me letters about their pregnancies and births and I couldn't believe the effort they made. I was really humbled.

Some of the gifts I was sent by companies did, however, leave me scratching my head. One gave me some prune juice and offered to send me crates more of the stuff, while another dispatched haemorrhoid cream!

I had one email which promised to 'look after Myleene's teeth and her baby's' – I thought, hang on, the baby is not even born yet. Another was an offer for a free baby first-aid course – which was brilliant. There were green nappies, dozens of pregnancy books

What's happening to your body – Week 17

You: Might already have had the first magical moment of feeling your baby moving around inside you. At first it will feel like very light and fluttery movement, known as 'quickening', which is almost indistinguishable from wind. As the weeks go on you will begin to recognise your baby's kicks, punches and rolls, although it will be several months before your partner can feel them too.

Your baby: Inside your tummy your 12cm baby – just a bit smaller than the width of this page – is moving about much more frequently and has probably discovered its first toy – the umbilical cord. The cord carries nutrients and oxygen from you to your baby while waste products travel in the opposite direction into your bloodstream and eventually into your kidneys.

and hundreds of toys.

Every day there was a different delivery. I couldn't help crying – but this time they were happy, joyful tears.

One of my earliest ever memories is visiting my aunt in the Philippines and getting an almighty smack from my mother for stealing the one toy that belonged to my seven cousins. They all slept in the same room and had nothing. It's something I will never forget.

I had worked so hard to be able to provide for my baby and now we were getting all this amazing stuff for free.

It was too much for us to keep. We decided to put it into three piles – one for us, one for my pregnant friends and one for a shelter near our house for single mothers and victims of abuse.

The generosity of people was incredible. There was one afternoon when Gray and I stood at our door as another truck disgorged more goodies for Rice.

'Rice is the luckiest baby in the world,' he told me. I couldn't disagree.

1 April 2007
Gray's Diary

Finally it's out. No more secrets. I'm over in Dublin for a lads' weekend. Came over to tell all my mates our news so have been pissed every night since I got here. Feel great today but forgot to tell a few people our news. Got a few texts from annoyed mates, but they'll be fine – if not, good luck to them! It will be easier on Leenie now. She has done so well to keep it a secret for all this time and to carry on working. Go out to the pub. Everyone is talking about the good news – feels great to be able to talk about it.

Week 18

The Week I Used a Made-up Word in Front of 200 Million People

In the days before I became pregnant I could memorise a page of script in five minutes, juggle six jobs with ease, retain a mountain of useless information and play whole concertos without a score. Now my house keys had to be colour-coded, I forgot the names of some of the most famous men in the world, I struggled to pronounce words and I could never remember what day it was.

Baby brain. If I hadn't suffered from it, I would have guffawed at the idea that it really existed; that pregnancy could make you forget or lose things and even change the way you speak.

But all I know is that something happened to me which meant I was just so much more stupid than I was before. Not only did I not know myself – I didn't even know where I was. Worst of all, for someone who did a lot of live television, I really struggled with my vocabulary.

The most cringeworthy example of this came while I was doing a live edition of my CNN show *The Screening Room*. Normally I just broadcast to Europe and Asia but this one was going around the world – to more than 200 million homes.

I was introducing a new actress and I wanted to say that this was her 'debut' film. But as I talked to the camera I realised that I had forgotten the word for debut. My mind was racing and I felt myself sweating but I just couldn't remember the word, which was on the tip of my tongue.

So, I'm ashamed to admit, I covered myself by making up a completely new word. 'And, of course, this is her nomora film . . .' I said as the cameraman gave me a strange look. I still cringe when I think of it.

It wasn't just words, but names, which also saw me caught out at live events.

On another occasion for CNN I kept referring to George Clooney as George Bush. Hello? I had to ask the producer to have a large board with names on as I evidently couldn't retain even the most simple information.

A few weeks later I was to make a huge mistake in front of 1,100 music fans when I introduced legendary composer and *Cabaret* actor Joel Grey by the wrong name at the rehearsal for the 'Night of A Thousand Voices' concert at the Albert Hall, and everyone gasped.

And my brain cells also caved in when I was presenting on *The People's Quiz* and actually managed to give away the answers in two of the questions: 'How many of the Seven Dwarfs had six beards? What did Yankee Doodle famously stick in his feather?' Doh! Doh! Doh!

When I went to present on BBC Four's '10 Best Elgar' show, in my brainwashed state I could only remember two of the pieces and ran out of descriptive words, calling every one of his works 'incredible'. I'm embarrassed at how bad I must have sounded.

As for remembering scripts – forget it. While I used to be able to do most of my reports in the first take, now it would need take after take, because I couldn't remember what I had just read.

My tip Unfortunately baby brain is one of those things you are just going to have to go with as there is no way of fighting it off. If you get stressed about it, you are likely to get even worse. Writing lists can definitely help but the only thing that will solve it is having your baby. And sometimes, even then, your baby brain can seem to actually get worse because of the sleep deprivation. But your old self will return – eventually.

Some of my jobs were relatively new – and I knew I was a far cry from the sharp presenter that I had been a few months earlier when they hired me. It was humiliating because I felt so rubbish – but there was nothing I could do. Luckily people were really understanding of my situation.

The worst thing about baby brain is that you know you have forgotten something – you just don't know what it was. The only way I could remember things at all was to write dozens of lists and to text things to myself.

But that did not help my general dippyness. At the Cannes Film Festival I mistakenly went into the men's toilets – bumping into Jerry Seinfeld, who thankfully had his trousers up. As I turned beetroot and had trouble explaining myself, he very kindly guided me to the ladies'.

I completely lost my car keys while, when we moved house, I was so confused about all the different keys that Gray had to colour-code them for me. I didn't know what had become of the strong, educated and work-mad woman I had been.

My doctor reckons baby brain exists because the baby drains all your energy and goodness from you. I have also heard it blamed on hormones and the fact that you are so sublimely occupied with your baby that you stop thinking about other things.

Certainly it was true that I was beginning to turn a bit gooey when it came to baby stuff. And then something happened which made me just as happy to talk about pink babygrows as I was about the latest movie star.

What's happening to your body – Week 18

You: Have probably gained at least half a stone by now and have a little bump. If you haven't already, it is time to get yourself some maternity clothes with waistbands that can stretch around or under your bump. Your breasts are continuing to change and grow, with milk ducts developing and veins becoming visible around your nipples. You may even start to leak colostrum, the early form of milk for your baby.

Your baby: Is now about 14cm long – the size of a banana. The development of the bones in its inner ear means that it can now sense sounds and hear you. It won't be able to detect your voice quite yet, but it can hear your heartbeat and very loud noises. You will also be able to hear your baby with the help of a special electronic advice called a Sonicaid. There is nothing more comforting to a worried mother than the loud galloping sound of your baby's heartbeat (but if you buy a machine for home use, don't forget that hearing the heartbeat depends on what position your baby is in).

6 April 2007
Gray's Diary

Leenie's birthday. I'm now starting to notice her body changing. Woke up this morning to these huge peaks in my face, which reminded me of the Alps. She has always had great boobs but now they are bigger than ever. I'm fine, though, I've got big hands. But I think for Leenie it's hard because of the extra weight and discomfort. Leenie keeps asking do I still find her sexy. If only she could get it into her mind that I'm closer to her now than ever. She is carrying our baby. I get up and make her breakfast in bed and give her her presents. She feels tired but happy.

Week 19

The Week Robert De Niro Stroked My Bump, Prompting Rice to Give a Kick

With me as its mama, Rice is likely to be both a huge film and music fan. So it was a pretty extraordinary day all round when my baby decided to give its first proper kick.

I had been having a bubbly feeling in my tummy for a couple of weeks. I can see why some people are confused about whether the sensation is actually wind or their little one moving about inside.

The first time it happened I wasn't sure myself. But after it kept on happening I realised that I could finally feel Rice moving about. I think the best way of describing it is as butterflies in your tummy – not the sick feeling you get when you are nervous, but of a proper little creature fluttering around inside.

There was no mistaking Rice's first kick, though.

I was in New York covering the Tribeca film festival for CNN and had just done one of the biggest interviews of my life – with film legend Robert De Niro. As I was waiting to meet him I was getting more and more nervous as all the other journalists in the room were talking about what a challenge he is, being so shy, he only ever gives monosyllabic answers.

My tip   *Those amazing kicks can often be shadowed by fear if you don't feel anything for a few hours. At this early stage, it is quite normal to even go for a whole day and not feel anything, because many of the movements are not yet strong enough. If you are worried at any point – and there will probably come a time when you will be – I found that waking baby up with a sugary treat while I lay in bed normally did the trick. But if you are still concerned by a lack of movement and are frightened that something is wrong, call your doctor for reassurance.*

So I couldn't believe that when I got to meet him he was charming, friendly and talkative.

He answered all my questions about his film, with bells on, but more importantly (for me, at least) he wished me luck with Rice and insisted on giving my bump a pat.

That evening, on the flight home to London, Rice had its say about such a momentous meeting with Hollywood royalty. I was watching the Beyonce Knowles film *Dreamgirls*, which I wasn't enjoying at all. But as soon as Beyonce started singing I felt a really strong kick. It was so amazing, like a wave going through my belly.

I started giggling and said, 'Hello, little baby,' as I patted my tummy. The producer on the seat next to me – who had been fast asleep – dreamily turned to me, asking, 'Did you want me?'

'I wasn't talking to you,' I laughed. It was the most incredible feeling. I was just gutted that I couldn't call Gray straightaway to tell him.

He was thrilled when I got to tell him although, disappointingly, it was several more months until he could feel the kicks himself. Feeling Rice for the first time made me realise how big and strong the baby was getting. It also made me feel a really powerful connection – like I had my little friend, who was a mini Gray, with me all the time.

I always loved getting kicked and poked and prodded about by Rice. And the kicks helped me identify the baby's personality – it was amazing but it already seemed to know its own mind, its own likes and dislikes.

Whenever I did a radio show I put a pair of headphones on my tummy so that Rice knew what I was doing. Rice appeared to love classical music – contemporary, which I approved of, Baroque, which was a surprise favourite, and big heavy players like Mozart, Brahms and Rachmaninov. The baby also loved pop – especially

What's happening to your body – Week 19

You: Are now five months pregnant. The top of your uterus probably almost reaches your belly button and will continue rising by about a centimetre a week. Your midwife will check this growth, known as the fundal height, during your appointments with her. With your tummy growing, your centre of gravity may have shifted so it is probably time to say goodbye to your highest heels.

Your baby: Is now about 15cm long from crown to rump – the length of a tube of toothpaste. This week the buds for your baby's permanent teeth will start forming behind the ones for its milk teeth. A protective substance called myelin also begins coating and insulating the baby's nerves – including the brain and spinal cord.

girls' voices – and happy music like albums by The Feeling and Duran Duran.

Favourite foods and drink included chocolate and Diet Coke – although it may have just been the caffeine that was causing the movements.

Rice would also kick when I got nervous – and it was like having a comforting best friend telling me, 'Don't worry, I'm here with you.'

And even though Gray could not yet feel Rice, he was about to become even more obsessed with talking to my tummy than I was.

Week 20

The Week We Discovered Rice Was a Girl

Choosing whether to find out the sex of your baby or not is another of those big pregnancy topics that everyone has an opinion on.

Most people were against it – saying it was nice to have an element of surprise. But I always felt that there is nothing more surprising than meeting your baby for the first time – even if you know it's a boy or a girl.

Everyone also wants to know which sex you would prefer. Of course I would always trot out the answer you have to give – that I just wanted it to be healthy. And of course I did. But, secretly, I was also hoping for a girl – and I was sure that I was having one.

The discussions about whether to find out whether we were having a girl or a boy went on for weeks. I was all for it. I had got sick of referring to Rice as 'it' – he or she was a little person, not an it.

And I couldn't see the point in waiting to see whether my instincts were right.

Gray ummm-ed and errr-ed about whether he wanted to know – although he was also desperate for a little girl. His friends all told him that it was nice to have an element of surprise, while his mother was adamantly against it. Finding out the sex is apparently

93

My tip Don't let other people sway you into making a decision on whether to find out your baby's sex. This is something that only you and your partner can decide. I don't regret finding out Rice was a girl for one second. It meant we could get everything we needed in pink! Before you do go through the whole big decision process, however, check that your hospital will tell you. Some districts refuse to tell parents what they are expecting, so you may have to wait to find out regardless of whether you wanted to know.

frowned upon in Ireland and she told him that we would be 'flying in the face of God'.

But I think her comments are what convinced Gray, being a contrary soul, to find out. He told his mother that the technology meant we already knew so much about Rice that finding out its sex only meant pointing the camera at a certain area.

Although I was sure I had a baby girl inside me everyone else – including Gray and my brother – thought Rice was a boy.

Everything, from the way I was carrying to the foods I was craving, seemed to indicate to total strangers that I was having a boy. I would frequently be stopped on the street by people telling me. I guess that shows you how accurate some of those old wives' tales are.

But the strangest thing happened on the evening before our twenty-week scan.

We were at Patrick Moore's party (yup, it's all rock and roll for us) with all these astronomers who were setting up their telescopes.

I have always been a fan of astronomy and had been studying it at Open University, so it was a thrill to be there. As usual, I needed to go to the toilet and went off to search for one.

I found the downstairs loo and there was a little old man sitting outside it. 'This is Patrick Moore's toilet,' he told me. 'No one else is allowed to use it but you as you are in the family way.'

When I came out, as I walked past him he said, 'It's a girl.' I whirled around and gave him a smile. 'Why did you say that?' I asked. 'Everyone else thinks it's a boy – cafeteria staff, people in the street, even my fiancé Gray.'

'When you find out you will remember this and you will remember me,' he said mysteriously. 'In all these years, I have never been wrong.'

He was slightly creepy in an all-seeing-prophet sort of way. And he was absolutely right.

At the scan the next day, there was the usual excitement tinged with anxiety, as we got to see our baby again.

Each time the doctor stopped to check the measurements and workings of Rice's organs, my heart missed a beat. Everything seemed fine – every time another limb or organ was looked at I would ask, 'Is that OK?' – but the doctor couldn't get the head measurements because Rice (as stubborn as her mother and camera shy as her father) refused to put her face in the right position.

The doctor was keen to get the profile shot before we did anything else, so for half an hour we prodded Rice and I jumped up and down. But nothing could convince her to move.

Finally, the doctor gave up but asked if we wanted to know the sex. I looked at Gray and said, 'It's up to you.' Without hesitating, he said, 'Yes.'

The next thing we knew, there was an image of a cute little

bottom and then the doctor told us we were having a girl.

I burst into tears while Gray grinned and yelled out, 'Yes! Yes!'

This time when we came out of the scan we were ecstatic. We were both flying off that afternoon – Gray to Ireland and me to Romania to film a video – but we felt closer than we had ever done before, imagining life with our daughter.

I also felt a great deal of relief that my instincts had been right. It made me realise that no one knew my little girl more than I did.

We phoned our families to tell them the news and there were more happy tears from them.

And the following week we got to see even more of our baby girl as we went for another scan to try and get those all-important head measurements. This time she moved her head obligingly for the doctor, kicked her leg high into the air, and had us all (my mum had come too, dressed in a smart hat for the occasion) giggling with joy.

What's happening to your body – Week 20

You: Are now officially halfway through your pregnancy. You will probably be offered another ultrasound scan to check your baby is developing properly and to see what position your placenta is in. You may also be able to find out what gender your baby is going to be – although finding out by ultrasound is not 100 per cent reliable. If all is progressing normally with your pregnancy, this is likely to be your last scan, so try and get your partner to attend with you.

Your baby: Now measures about 16.5cm – the length of a tall glass – and is steadily gaining weight. A greasy white substance called vernix caseosa begins to cover its delicate skin to protect it from the amniotic fluid. Some babies may still be covered in it if they are born prematurely.

The doctor listened to her heartbeat and pronounced it to be 'strong like a tiger'. Such happiness.

Of course, the fact that I knew the sex did not stop people trying to guess. Some friends even convinced me to do the ring test – when you tie a ring onto a piece of string and see whether it circles (boy) or goes from side to side (girl). I did it twice and there was a different answer both times.

Meanwhile, before even asking me if I had found out, people would still come up to me in the street and tell me, 'It's a boy, definitely a boy.' A lady who works in the canteen at the BBC would say it to me every week. I didn't have the heart to tell them the truth.

We had found out we were having a baby girl – but now our big decision was going to be what to call her.

26 April 2007
Gray's Diary

Today I'm over the moon to find out we are having a little girl. I can't believe it – I'm going to have a mini panda (my name for Leenie). She will be beautiful like her mammy. She will be cherished. This is the best news. We are so lucky to have this happen to us. Hurry up, Rice, can't wait to meet you.

Week 21

The Week I Wanted to Call My Daughter Vegas

My hormones had calmed down, my sickness had disappeared and Gray and I were getting on fabulously. Until, that is, we started discussing what name to give our daughter.

It was an absolute minefield. I thought I knew Gray, and I had always believed we had similar taste. But we really struggled to find anything to agree on.

A name is so important – in a way you are creating a personality just by what you call your child.

One of my friends told me a fun way of choosing a name to pass the taste barrier: it should be a name that would fit the life of a lawyer, a rock star and a poet. I have to admit that in some of my more desperate moments, however, I was coming up with names that broke all the rules.

My favourite names were grand ones with lots of syllables like Anastasia, or ancient ones I knew from astronomy like Callisto and Persophone. With names like that, I reasoned, you could only be destined for great things. But Gray thought they sounded like Austro-Hungarian princesses and didn't like them at all.

He wasn't much help, though. He knew the names he didn't like but the only ones he could come up with were of famous women that he fancied: Halle (as in Berry), Helena (as in Christiansen) and

Rihanna (after the R&B singer).

One early name we did agree on was Rose, but then we realised that as Gray has an Auntie Rose there would be lots of politics about why we had named our child after her and none of the other aunties.

We both also liked Irish-sounding names like Alannah and Oisean – but when Gray said them it sounded like he was sneezing. My father was insistent that we call her Angelina – but neither of us were that keen – as my middle name is already Angela.

In desperation I started thinking about more unusual names. I met a lovely gay couple who'd had a terrible time trying to have their kids – who were called Vegas and Arizona. It was such a heart-warming story that I fell in love with the name Vegas. But when I told Gray he looked at me like I was mad and said there was no way he was going to name our daughter after a showgirl.

Looking back, I can see he was right.

One of the few names that we both quite liked was Ava. We had been toying with calling her after my mother, Evangelista, but my

My tip Names – another of those big subjects that everyone seems to have an opinion on. It is a big deal, as in a way you are determining the way your child will be perceived in the world. Try not to get carried away in the moment like I did with Vegas – and think about how that name will fit your baby as they grow up in the world. You will be very lucky if everyone you talk to likes the name you have chosen – the most important people to be happy with it should be you and your partner.

brother had already bagsied that, so we had been thinking about Eva and Ava.

And then, weirdly, two of the people we were closest to mentioned the name Ava on the same day. I was on the phone to Lauren and she was saying what a beautiful name it was and how it had this glamour attached to it from Ava Gardner. Then, just a few hours later, Gray's sister also suggested Ava.

The shortlist was Ava, Helena and Alannah.

What's happening to your body – Week 21

You: Probably gave up lying on your front some weeks ago and it may now be time to stop lying on your back for too long. Sleeping or resting on your back puts the full weight of your bump onto your spine and the vein that transports blood from your lower body to your heart. As well as making you feel a bit dizzy, it can increase the risk of backache, haemorrhoids and poor digestion. Try and get into the habit of lying on your left side, as it will maximise the flow of blood and nutrients to your placenta – although do not worry if you wake up and find yourself on your back. If your bump is already making you feel uncomfortable when you are trying to sleep, put a pillow between your legs and under your bump. You can also buy special maternity pillows which can be used later on for feeding your baby.

Your baby: Is about 18.5cm long – as tall as an aubergine. It now has tiny fingernails and groomed eyebrows and its ears have developed enough to hear your conversations. Now is a good time to encourage Daddy to talk and sing to your bump. You can play your favourite music and even read it stories – studies have shown that young babies seem to recognise books which were read to them in utero, while your voice can have an instant calming effect.

When we put it to Rice, Ava came up tops every time. Whenever we suggested what names to call her we always got a kick when we said Ava – it was uncanny.

There was one other name that we had both fallen in love with, and one that Rice also seemed to like – Bailey. Our only problem was that it was a boy's name, but I still wanted it.

1 May 2007
Gray's Diary

Since the second scan I have been speaking to Leenie's little bump. I was told that Rice can hear me so I want her to know my voice straightaway. Every morning and every night I talk to her and when Leenie is sleeping I wake up and tell Rice all about me and her mama and the rest of her family. I tell her how we are all dying to meet her. It's mad, I could talk to her bump for hours. I just hope she can really hear me because I have been talking so much. If not, I have been set up and this is a joke on me – ha-ha. Anyway, I like doing it, it makes me happy to think she can hear her daddy.

Week 22

The Week Sex Went Off the Menu

It was sex that got you into this little adventure but for some couples making love goes completely out the window during pregnancy.

Other couples are at it like rabbits until the labour and it is apparently the best way of inducing labour once you are overdue.

Like many of my friends, we were somewhere in between.

In my first trimester I was feeling so tired and sick that the last thing I normally fancied was sex. Going to bed alone to sleep was much more appealing. Then there was the fact that my boobs were so painful that if anyone came near them it felt like they were brandishing a hot poker and I would jump a mile.

But once I started feeling better in my second trimester I felt curvier than ever before and really sensual. And I fancied Gray like mad. He was the man who had made me pregnant – I felt like we were an uber-couple who could take on the world. It was fantastic for a few weeks.

And then two things happened: my bump grew and we found out we were having a girl.

By five months your bump is likely to be hard to miss. If you do continue with the bedroom activities you can find that it does actually sometimes become more *Carry On . . .* than *9½ Weeks*. So be prepared for lots of giggles.

Once you get your bump, many men can become a little scared. They can be frightened of hurting the baby, scared the baby will hear them and also worried about hurting you. They can also be totally terrified by the idea of leaking breasts, which happened to at least one friend of mine when she had an orgasm.

And once your partner has seen the baby moving about on the scan and may even, like us, have discovered the sex, they can be even more freaked.

If your partner no longer wants sex it can make you feel unattractive and unloved.

It's hard enough to feel sexy when you are a pregnant woman – you definitely feel like men look at you differently. Although I

What's happening to your body – Week 22

You: Have probably gained over a stone now and the weight will start to climb more steadily as your baby gets bigger. From this week you may start to experience painless contractions called Braxton Hicks contractions. They feel like a squeezing sensation as your uterus practises for labour. Some women experience them for weeks before their labour, others just a few hours before the big moment and some never get them. Braxton Hicks contractions are not painful – so if you are having painful contractions you need to contact your doctor.

Your baby: Measures about 19.5cm from crown to rump – the size of the height of this page – and now weighs almost a pound. Its skin is wrinkled because it does not have much fat and is opaque, but over the next few weeks it will gain weight and the skin will thicken. A black tarry goo called meconium is beginning to accumulate in its bowels from many of the things it has swallowed in the amniotic fluid. This will usually appear as the baby's first poo.

revelled in my new curves I know that for a lot of men pregnancy is a no-go area.

I had this one incident around the five-month mark when I was getting on a plane and there were three guys behind me. One of them gave a wolf whistle but when I turned around the effect was instantaneous. Their jaws dropped and they didn't know where to look. When I saw them later at the baggage pick-up they wouldn't even look at me.

Gray did his best to make me feel loved and attractive but there was a part of me that knew I appeared different in his eyes because I was carrying his baby – I was no longer just his partner but now the mother of his unborn child.

But I was also discovering there were upsides to having a huge bump – it seemed the world's most gorgeous men couldn't take their hands off me.

My tip When relations have been as strained as they were between Gray and me after all of my hormonal behaviour, sex is a great way to remind yourselves why you are a couple. It is certainly possible throughout pregnancy and I know plenty of friends who continued for the whole nine months. But then I also have friends who believed 'three is a crowd' from the start and abstained completely.

I would say, like everything to do with pregnancy, you have to do what is right for you and your partner.

It is worth remembering that fears of hurting the baby are almost always misplaced (although doctors often caution against it if you have a history of miscarriage). It is well cushioned inside its amniotic sac, while the uterus is sealed off by a thick, mucous plug (and if reading that doesn't put your man off sex, I don't know what will).

Your baby will also have no idea of what you are doing – or any memory of it.

But you can't blame your man for looking at you differently – you are different.

Week 23

The Week When Johnny Depp, Brad Pitt, George Clooney and Matt Damon All Insisted on Touching My Bump and Talking Babies (Swoon)

There is obviously something about a bump that makes men and women – especially if they are parents themselves – go all gooey. They want to touch the bump, they want to talk baby names, they want to tell you all about their children. They want to share with you how exciting it is in the parent club. And most of all, they want to give you lots of advice.

And I was discovering that celebrities, even world-famous A-list multimillionaire ones, are no different. I might have lost my sex appeal but I had mummy-to-be appeal and it was an amazing icebreaker.

I started May meeting one of my all time heart-throbs: Johnny Depp, who was in London for the latest *Pirates of the Caribbean* junket. I had a whole list of questions in front of me but could barely get a word in edgeways as he was far more interested in finding out how far gone I was, how I was feeling, whether I knew the sex, etc., etc.

'Your children are the most precious thing you can ever have,' he told me.

When it came to talking about the film our conversation was – ironically – far more laboured. But as I went to leave he insisted on giving my bump a pat and said: 'Give your baby a kiss from Uncle Johnny.' Hell, yes!

He was the first of a long list of my favourite men that Rice was to prove an instant hit with.

A few weeks later I was covering the Cannes Film Festival where *Ocean's 13* was being premiered. I had tonnes of questions for Brad, George and Matt but they were far more interested in finding out about Rice and helping me come up with names.

George suggested Fionnula and Buella while Brad said Mary. Matt, who insisted that he be the first to have a rub, said I should call her Isabella after his own daughter. I couldn't believe how being pregnant both relaxed and excited everyone around me – especially dads. It particularly seemed to bring out their protective qualities.

So after Robert de Niro having a pat a few weeks ago, Rice had now been touched by the gorgeous quartet of Johnny, Brad, George and Matt.

And when I met Sir Paul McCartney at the Classical BRITs, he was also eager to feel my bump. He was up for Album of the Year and asked if he could have a rub for luck. It obviously did the trick as he went on to win it.

Later on in the evening we were talking together when someone came up to invite me to a record company bash. Sir Paul looked at me very seriously and said, 'Myleene, I think you should go home and get some rest.' I did as I was told!

Celebrity advice came from far and wide. Earl Spencer, who said he'd done all the night feeds for his children, told me to sleep while I could as I would need it. Suzi Quatro told me to never wear heels. Geri Halliwell said having a girl was the best as you could dress her up as a little doll.

Some of the strangest pieces of advice were about the birth itself. 'Moo like a cow,' one stylist told me. 'It will relax you and the baby.'

When I was on GMTV Lorraine Kelly suddenly told me to: 'Keep your shoulders down,' causing me to instantly relax my shoulders. 'No, not now, silly, when you are in labour. It's a tip the Queen's obstetrician told me.' To this day, I am not sure why. I must remember to ask her!

And it wasn't just the celebrities. Everyone I met – whether on the street or at a red-carpet premiere – had some advice or other.

Although it was lovely to know that people cared, and some of it was useful, the mountain of uninvited advice I was getting began to irritate me, especially as it sometimes seemed like people were criticising me. I got sick of people – including my own family – telling me how I should and should not behave.

When I was on *The One Show* there was plenty of concern from viewers that I would give myself varicose veins by crossing my legs.

'Myleene – please stop crossing your legs, it's worrying my mum so much,' said one typical email. 'She's worried that you'll end up with varicose veins on your legs! Not a pretty sight.'

Another said: 'I can't bear to look at you as you always sit with your legs crossed. It's so bad for you – ask any midwife.'

I tried to stop crossing my legs but it was habit. And when I asked my doctor about it he said that it was an old wives' tale and I shouldn't worry. He told me that varicose veins are more normally down to genes than leg crossing.

My tip It is impossible to be angry with people for giving you unwanted advice by the truckload as they are only trying to help. I suggest you grit your teeth, smile diplomatically and say thank you. Everyone has a need to share their own experiences with you and, as per usual, the advice can often be contradictory. But before you know it you will be a mummy too and you may find yourself biting your tongue before becoming the advice-giver.

I would get advice that I was eating too much or too little. One fitness freak – who had recently become a mother herself – told my manager: 'Myleene is clearly enjoying eating for two. She's going to end up regretting it.'

Perfect strangers were sometimes the worst. One man came up to me in the street and said: 'You're too big!' When I shot back, 'How big am I supposed to be?' he replied: 'It depends how far gone you are.' Right, so he didn't know how far along I was but had decided I was too big!

Others would just touch my tummy without asking. I hated that. How would they like it if I touched theirs?

Lots of people seemed to want to tell Gray and me what I should be doing for my pregnancy. Many of our friends were aghast that we had decided against attending any antenatal classes. We did do a baby first-aid course but neither of us thought I really needed to learn how to breathe – I was a trained singer after all.

As far as I was concerned, women gave birth for centuries

without going to antenatal classes and I knew that my midwife and doctor would be there to talk me through everything.

But our decision seemed to really upset people. One night Gray rang me from the pub – all his friends had ganged up on him to try and force us to go to a group.

My sister, who doesn't have any children herself, also got very distressed that I had decided I didn't want to use a TENS machine. I don't know why she was so obsessed with it, but she tried really hard to get me to buy one.

What's happening to your body – Week 23

You: May be experiencing common pregnancy symptoms such as bleeding gums when you brush your teeth. Blame the hormones (again!) which are making your gums inflamed. If you are worried you can see the dentist free of charge while you are pregnant. Another place you may be bleeding from is your nose. The hormones are also increasing blood flow to the mucous membranes in your nose, causing them to swell. As well as frequent nosebleeds these can cause nasal stuffiness and even sinusitis. Saline sprays can help, as can using a humidifier and nasal strips. But if you have sinusitis you may need to see your doctor, who will prescribe you antibiotics.

Your baby: Now measures 20cm – about the size of a male hand – and its face looks fully formed with distinct lips, a button nose and developing eyes – although they do not yet have any colour. Its brain is also growing and will continue to expand until your baby is five years old. Its reproductive system is also becoming formed. Girls already have their uterus, ovaries and vagina while primitive sperm have formed in the testes of the boys. If your baby were born now it would have nearly a 20 per cent chance of survival – in another week that will have doubled to 44 per cent.

Almost everyone I knew told me that I needed to get some routine in my life. But I was hoping that the baby would fall into my life rather than my life being led by her.

But that is not to say I didn't take some of the advice on board – so many people told me the same things that I knew they had to be right.

'Always communicate with each other' was one that I could understand, particularly as I knew how bad things had got because of my hormones.

'Talk to other recent mothers' was another – as the advice had changed so much since my mother had me, on everything from what position the baby should sleep in to how often it should feed.

But the one that became my mantra was 'Mummy knows best' – at the end of the day you have to trust your instincts.

Week 24

The Week I Posed Naked for a Magazine

I would say that, like many women, I have a love–hate relationship with my body. And for most of my life it has been intense dislike. I'm not a naturally skinny girl and since I was a teenager my weight has yo-yoed.

At the peak of Hear'Say's fame I was a size 14 and the band's management were constantly on at me to lose weight. When the band finished I had shrunk to a small size 8. But even then, when fashion designers were enthusing about how 'fabulous' I looked, I felt uncomfortable and unhappy – and Gray hated my body, calling me Boney-M.

So for me, one of the most amazing things about pregnancy was that I felt truly comfortable with my body for the first time.

Yes, I was putting on what seemed to be half a stone every time I saw the doctor. Yes, my boobs were huge, my thighs had expanded and I had what Lauren and I termed 'armulite' on my upper arms (how had I put on weight there?).

But my body was making a baby and I felt fabulous.

I would never have agreed to go naked on the front cover of a magazine before my pregnancy but when *Glamour* magazine asked me if I would 'do a Demi' (after Demi Moore's famous pregnancy pose for *Vanity Fair*) I thought it was a fantastic idea.

It all started as a bit of a joke. I was on the judging panel of GMTV's High Street Awards with the *Glamour* editor Jo Elvin and we got quite friendly. One lunch time she was telling me she was having a nightmare trying to choose a celebrity to be on the front of the magazine's August issue. 'At this rate, I'm going to have to ask you to do a Demi for me,' she said.

I didn't think anything more about it, but the next day my publicist phoned me and said, 'What's all this about you going naked for *Glamour*?'

It wasn't something I had thought about before but I immediately agreed and just a few weeks later I was posing in front of dozens of people at the shoot with just a G-string to preserve my modesty.

It was one of the nicest shoots I had ever been on. Practically everyone there was a parent so we talked babies all day. When I got hot flushes they all understood what I was going through. And I didn't feel embarrassed scoffing my usual fish and chips.

And I felt proud of my body. It's the first time I have ever done any sort of modelling and not felt compelled to suck my tummy in. I had the same experience a few weeks later when I was hosting the Miss Scotland competition and for once didn't feel fat and

My tip Pregnancy can be so difficult that sometimes it is hard to enjoy what is happening to your body. So take time to revel in your curves, enjoy the changes that are happening to your body and think about how wonderful you are – you are making a baby. How incredible is that!

ungainly next to all the aspiring beauty queens.

In fact, I was revelling in my curves and became quite vain about them! If I caught a glimpse of my profile while shopping I would stop, have a proper look and rub my belly. My boobs might have expanded to a size 32E and none of my trousers fitted but being pregnant meant I was 100 per cent happy with the way I looked.

It wasn't just that I didn't have to suck in my belly. It was an incredible time: my body was creating a baby. When you are pregnant you realise how awe-inspiring nature is. It's incredible how your body knows to create a placenta, how your bones know to soften to help with the labour, how you breathe deeper to take in more oxygen.

Getting pregnant can be hard and sustaining a pregnancy just as hard – in a way both are miracles in themselves.

But I think that in this country people are split into two groups

What's happening to your body – Week 24

You: May notice faint red streaks across your tummy, hips, backside and breasts – the dreaded stretch marks. Although there are dozens of creams and oils on the market to combat them, many scientists believe that whether they appear or not comes down to genes. If they are going to appear, it will normally be around now. Although they are impossible to get rid of totally, they will eventually fade. The creams and oils can, however, help with another pregnancy problem – itchy skin caused by it stretching to accommodate your growing figure.

Your baby: Measures 21cm from crown to rump, as big as a small doll, and if it stretched its legs out too it would reach the end of your 30cm ruler. Its taste buds are formed, so if you are enjoying lots of sweets and chocolate it will be too.

– they either celebrate pregnancy or treat it like an illness. The *Glamour* shoot was a celebration of pregnancy and I felt empowered.

However, not everyone saw it that way. Even my mother was a little bit shocked when I told her – she literally couldn't speak. But she absolutely loved the pictures when they appeared, as did Gray.

The front cover seemed to polarise opinion – which to me summed up how different people see pregnancy in Britain. I got lots of letters and emails saying how wonderful it was but there were quite a few which said how it was disgusting – pregnant women should be hiding their bumps not showing them off.

I was surprised that a lot of the angry letters came from women who presumably would have preferred it if I had disappeared into confinement as soon as I had discovered I was pregnant. It made me annoyed that people – especially women who had children themselves – seemed to think pregnant women should be hidden from view.

19 May 2007
Gray's Diary

Went to visit Leenie's mam and dad's for dinner. Takes forever to get Leenie out of the house. I'm used to being on time. At work I'm a 100mph person. But since the baby I'm starting to chill a bit and I know I can't rush her. I know she is doing her best. I stand by the door and say nothing. Just when she is ready to leave I know what she will do — go for a wee. I have never seen someone go to the toilet so many times. I should have bought shares in Andrex toilet paper as we go through so many rolls. Finally we get in the car and off we go but, trust me, I have planned the route so I know where we can go for toilet breaks. And the car is always stocked with water, orange juice, apples (Pink Lady only), wet wipes and chocolates. We're ready for war!

Week 25

The Week We Decided We Had Better Move Nearer My Parents

I am sure I am not the first pregnant woman to suddenly reassess her own mother as she prepares to become a mum herself.

As my bond with Rice grew by the day I truly realised what the unconditional love of being a parent really means. And I began to understand how much my mum loved me. Having brought up three children without any help at all, I now saw that she was an extraordinary goddess. And I felt pretty awful about all my bad behaviour as a teenager and how ungrateful I had been.

And then she did, perhaps, the biggest thing for me of all – she volunteered to be my granny nanny.

Gray and I had already started discussing what we were going to do about childcare once Rice finally made her arrival. We were both keen for me to return to work but did not want to have to rely on a stranger to help look after our baby. We were planning to share the childcare between the two of us.

But my parents had different plans in mind.

'No, that's not going to happen,' my mother told us. 'She's going to be with her *lola* (Philippine for granny).' I told her I couldn't possibly expect her to look after Rice and come into work

117

My tip It may feel too early to be thinking about childcare but if you are planning to go back to work quite quickly, then it is something you should at least be contemplating. Some popular nurseries have waiting lists of up to a year – and they even allow you to put your name down when you are still pregnant. If you are considering a child minder or nanny, speak to friends in the area to see if they have any recommendations. And if you are as lucky as me to have hands-on parents who agree to help out, shower them with kisses and cuddles and make sure they know how much you appreciate them.

with me but she put her foot down – as did my father, who told us that there was no way we were going to let anyone else look after Rice.

It was a done deal – they had clearly thought about it a lot. And we were overwhelmed by their kindness. I was also so happy because it would mean that our daughter would really get to know her grandparents.

I never really knew mine – my mother's parents lived in the Philippines and I only met them once or twice while my father's mother was Austrian and, although she lived in Wales and we used to see her at Christmas, there was a language barrier which meant we were never close.

It was and is brilliant of my parents to agree to look after Rice. But it did mean that we needed to reassess our living arrangements.

We lived in a flat on the Thames in the southeast of London while my parents were quite far to the north of the capital. Gray had been working like a horse to turn our mezzanine level into a nursery and we had not thought much further ahead than bringing Rice home to it.

But as spring approached and the sun came out and I missed, yet again, having a garden we also started thinking about the reality of being parents. We thought about how we would soon be outgrowing our little flat and also about the long journey either we or my parents were going to have to make.

I didn't want to push Gray into moving near my parents as he had lived in south London since leaving Dublin at eighteen and crossing the Thames can be a lot like crossing the Rubicon. But I was secretly hoping that he would come around to my way of thinking.

It helped that we had already started seeing a lot more of my family. Even though the baby had not yet arrived it already seemed that we had both become closer to our parents and siblings. We are both very lucky that we come from stable happy homes and it felt brilliant that we were now going to be one huge family.

Gray's mother was full of good advice for things like morning sickness. And while at first Gray's sister did seem to be wondering whether I was quite ready for motherhood, as a relatively new mum herself she was brilliant for her many words of wisdom.

My brother and sister were getting really excited about their niece and I saw more of them than I had for years. And while my father appeared to be struggling with being called Grandpa – he thought it was an insult rather than a statement of fact – he was the one who really persuaded us that my mum could help us look after the baby.

My family even held a special baby shower – which was called her 'baby rinse' – in which each member made pledges to Rice with promises ranging from 'covering her in kisses and cuddles' to 'teaching her karate'. I felt so lucky to have such an incredible unit around me.

We already spent lots of weekends at my parents' house talking about the baby and – after considering the fact that if we were going to do this journey every week we could be facing a two-hour commute on the North Circular – Gray was persuaded to start looking for a house in north London.

I am rather lucky that Gray is obsessed by property and I was able to leave most of the house hunting in his capable hands. After several frustrating weeks he found the perfect house – the only problem was that it wasn't built yet.

What's happening to your body – Week 25

You: As your baby moves up your abdomen – it is now over the top of your belly button – you may be suffering from heartburn, which is caused both by the hormonal changes in your body and the physical ones. Hormones relax the valve that separates the oesophagus from the stomach, allowing acid to escape, while your growing baby pushes up stomach acids to cause the burning sensation. You should try to limit your intake of spicy foods and citrus fruits and eat regular small meals rather than three big ones. Several over-the-counter remedies can also be taken by pregnant women to get rid of the pain, but talk to your doctor first.

Your baby: Now measures 23cm, the diameter of a plate, and its lungs are almost developed enough to breathe. If it were born now your baby would have a 70 per cent chance of survival.

The plot, just fifteen minutes away from where my parents live, was where an old house had been pulled down. A developer was just about to start work on it so because he hadn't done anything yet it meant that we could have it built exactly as we wanted. It was Gray's dream.

The only problem was that it would not be ready until November at the earliest – but Rice was due in September and we had to sell our flat.

I felt more than a bit stressed when we realised we were going to be without a home for the first few months of our baby's life. I really appreciated the fact that we were lucky enough to be building our own house but, like all new mothers, I would have liked to nest – to make my baby's room all pink and perfect and to have a sparkling clean home to bring her to. Now I didn't even have a home to bring her to at all.

And when our flat sold much quicker than we could have hoped (just six weeks before my due date), the pressure was really on – we then had six days to find a flat to rent and pack everything up.

26 May 2007
Gray's Diary

Watched a Steve Martin movie called Cheaper By The Dozen 2. It was so weird because as we are about to have a baby we are seeing it in a totally different way. I really felt for the dad, what it's like to be a father or mother — this is all ahead of me. I can't wait but there are some bits I'm not looking forward to: the day your little girl grows up and some spotty teen calls around to take her out. I know it's going to happen, and I know what men are like — I was one of the worst. So to think I will have to go through this kills me. I remember when I was younger and my mam and dad said, 'Wait until you have your own kids, you will know what we mean.' 'Yeah, yeah,' I used to say to them, 'I will be different when I'm a dad.' And now when I think about it, I know I will be a lot worse. My poor girl, she doesn't know what's waiting for her in the future! Any spotty teen tries it on with her and he will have to get through me first.

Week 26

The Week My Doctor Told Me to Stop Eating So Many Doughnuts

I was loving my bump and feeling gloriously sensual with all my curves.

But not everybody saw it that way. By the time I was six months pregnant I had already put on three stone. I needed to eat to keep both the nausea and exhaustion at bay (at least that was what I was telling myself, although both had subsided significantly) and I was enjoying the chance of being able to eat what I wanted.

Every time I went to see Dr Mason he would say, 'OK, pop on the scales and let's make sure you're eating well.' I would pop on the scales – I would probably have put on about another seven pounds – and it was obvious I was eating well.

When I reached eleven stone I jokingly said, 'Wow, I really am putting on a lot of weight,' hoping for a reassuring comment about how it was necessary to keep piling the pounds on.

So I was quite surprised when he shot back: 'Well, you don't have to eat quite so many doughnuts. You can find the weight catching up with you.'

He was right. I was enjoying my pregnancy and the excuse to eat as many biscuits as I liked. And I knew I should be eating more

My tip The important thing when you are pregnant is that you are happy. A happy relaxed mummy makes a happy relaxed baby. So if you are feeling fat and bloated then the best thing to do is to make time for yourself and to make yourself feel better. For some people that might mean doing a bit of exercise, for others it will be a nice facial or a massage. A beauty treatment is a fantastic way to treat yourself when you are feeling tired and heavy – and there are plenty of companies which specialise in treatments you can do at home. Or you might even want to get a spray tan. If you are planning to get yourself a beauty treatment I would advise always phoning ahead to make sure they cater for pregnant women. And if you want to buy a treatment in the chemist make sure you read the small print – the last thing you want is to be relaxing with a nice face mask only to discover you should have checked with your doctor before putting it on.

salad and less chocolate. But, but, but. I really did find that carbohydrates helped with the energy. I really did find that I craved ginger biscuits. And I really did need my baked potatoes with cheese. I was working so hard that I couldn't possibly survive on carrot juice alone.

I also should have been exercising. Every other pregnancy book you will read will tell you about how you should be getting fit, doing gentle exercise and preparing your body for labour. But I am sure I am not alone when I confess that although I had great plans to exercise – particularly as I had felt so fit and healthy after the jungle – I was generally too tired. Being in bed was much more appealing.

I have never been a massive gym-goer but I have always kept fit with skipping and kick boxing. They were, obviously, both out, being high impact and with lots of potential for accidents.

Swimming, walking and pregnant yoga are the three main exercises that most health professionals agree pregnant women should be doing.

I have never been one for yoga or Pilates. When I have tried out classes in the past, instead of concentrating on my breathing I would be doing shopping lists in my head. So that didn't appeal.

Gray would try and drag me to the gym with him and occasionally we would go swimming together. It did feel fantastic being in the pool – I would feel light and buoyant – sensations I had actually forgotten. But I always found it a bit of a drag once I got out of the pool – I would feel heavy once again and then I had to dry my hair and get the smell of chlorine off me.

I did try and do as much walking as I could. I even used to – occasionally – walk up lots of flights of stairs. I became more aware about how I could walk from job to job and would occasionally even go for walks at the weekends.

It was far from the twenty minutes a day that most manuals advise but I was exhausted and I chose to keep rested rather than drive myself mad with exercise.

So the only exercise that I would do rigidly was my pelvic floors. I didn't know much about them before I got pregnant but once you are expecting a baby – and even more when you have had one – you need to be doing these exercises regularly.

It's hard to work out the benefits and often you don't even know if you are doing them correctly. But I've heard enough people say that I will be grateful for doing them when I reach fifty to make me continue.

The pelvic floor is the muscle that runs between your legs to the base of your spine, holding your bladder, uterus and bowel in place. Pregnancy and labour can weaken them and if you don't do your exercises you can become incontinent.

Hmmm, that word was enough to frighten me into doing them pretty constantly. I followed the advice that you could work out what the muscle was when you try and halt doing a wee mid-flow.

My sister told me that one way of doing the exercises is to imagine your pelvic floor is a lift. You go up one floor and hold, go up another floor (pulling in tighter) and hold, and then go up another floor before going back down to the start. The analogy became a memory trigger for me – every time I got in a lift I would do my pelvic floor exercises. Well, it was a good excuse not to use the stairs.

My weight gain had gone to my thighs and arms as well as my tummy. It meant that I felt uncomfortable wearing even maternity jeans as I thought they made me look short and stout.

When it came to maternity clothes I was very lucky that I had M&S, who sent me their entire range. But I wasn't allowed to wear their clothes on the BBC for my nightly evening show *The One Show* as it was viewed as endorsement.

I know there is a lot more choice for fashionable maternity wear than there was a few years ago but I still really struggled to find good clothes that I wanted to wear. I found a few shops with really nice outfits – Crave, Mamas and Papas, Isabella Oliver and the Homme Mummy range were my favourites with clothes that clung to my bump – but I was generally disappointed with many of the maternity ranges.

I was lucky, however, that the fashion in the summer I was pregnant was for long maxi dresses and full smocks. I was wearing normal clothes in a size 14 from shops like Zara, French Connection and Warehouse right up until the day I gave birth. (For a full list of my favourite maternity shops see page 204.)

When it comes to dressing with a bump my advice would be to show it off rather than try and hide it. And although maternity wear can still be disappointing, there are other ways to make you look good.

I have already described how I carried on having my hair coloured with a diluted solution. And from my second trimester my hair felt better than ever as it was thick and shiny.

My skin had recovered from the pimples of the first trimester. Even Gray, who I'm sure is a secret frustrated beautician, struggled to find any spots to pick when I was sleeping next to him (one of his more endearing habits, I don't think).

I got given a few presents of massages and facials especially for pregnancy, which were all wonderful. You can often have your normal beauty treatment but beauticians take out the essential oils because it is not known what impact they can have on pregnancy.

I would also massage oil on myself every day, as I was terrified of getting stretch marks. Some people say whether you get the marks is down to your genes rather than anything else but I wasn't taking any chances. Gray used to say it was like sleeping next to an oil slick.

And if in doubt, and in need of a good pick-me-up, you can always fake it. It had been a rubbish summer so I didn't have my usual tan and I received a few letters asking if I was OK as I was looking 'a bit peaky'.

Obviously I didn't want to go on the sun bed so I decided to get a spray tan. When I got to a salon, however, the assistant refused to do it, showing me paperwork which said the now familiar line that pregnant women should not have it done without talking to their doctor first.

I had been waiting half an hour to get to the front of the queue but didn't want to proceed without knowing the full facts so asked her, 'Look, if I phone my doctor and he OKs it, will you let me have the spray tan?'

When she agreed, I phoned up my doctor's surgery. I planned to only speak to the nurse there – thinking that I couldn't possibly bother my doctor with something so ridiculous. But before I had even blurted out why I had rang, the nurse put me through to Dr Mason.

Feeling rather embarrassed to be phoning him over something so silly – it was the first time I had ever phoned with a question – I blustered, 'Erm, erm, doctor, erm, is it OK if I have a spray tan?' Suppressing a laugh he said, 'I don't see why not – may I enquire what colour you are planning to go?

What's happening to your body – Week 26

You: With your growing bump, heartburn, back ache, need to go to the toilet and a myriad of other pregnancy symptoms, a restful night's sleep may now be a thing of the past. You may also be having vivid nightmares as your subconscious plays out your fears about what is to come. Gentle yoga and meditation before bed can really help with pregnancy insomnia. Other remedies include drinking a glass of warm milk, munching on a piece of celery (it contains a compound called phthalide which relaxes muscles), and cherries (which induce the sleep hormone melatonin).

Your baby: Now measures 25cm, the length of a size-6 shoe. Your baby's lungs can now inhale and exhale. It will respond to touch and if you shine a light on your abdomen it will turn its head, an early sign of the functioning of the optic nerve.

I was too exhausted to do anything but sleep once I got to bed.

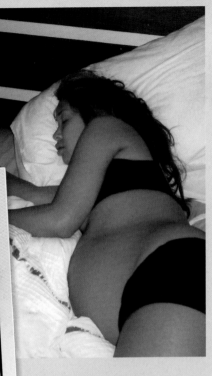

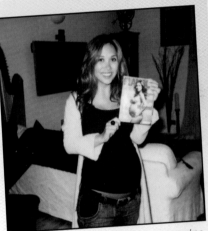

I rushed out to get *Glamour* magazine and was really happy about flying the flag for mamas by posing naked on the cover.

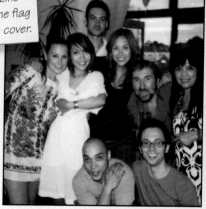

Baby rinse: M (Don's girlfriend), Jessie, Jake (her husband), Dad, Mama, cousin John and Don.

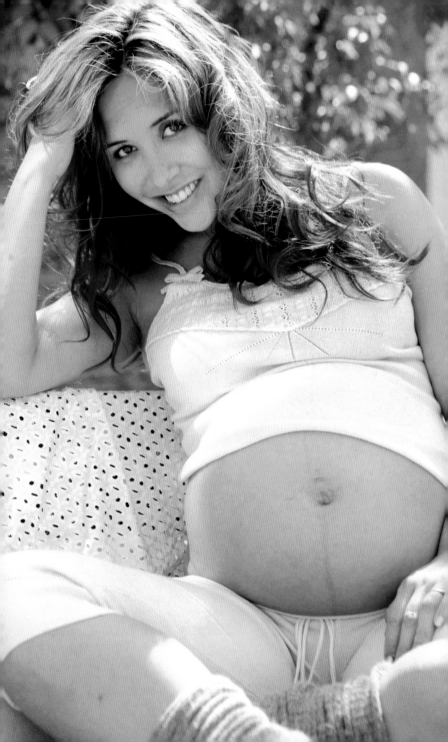

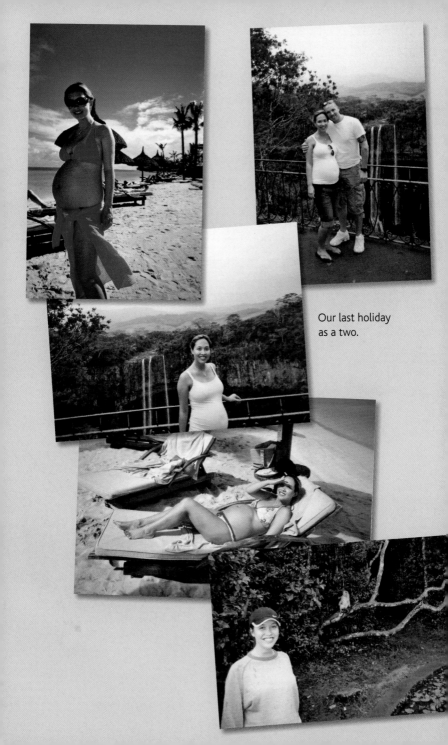

Our last holiday
as a two.

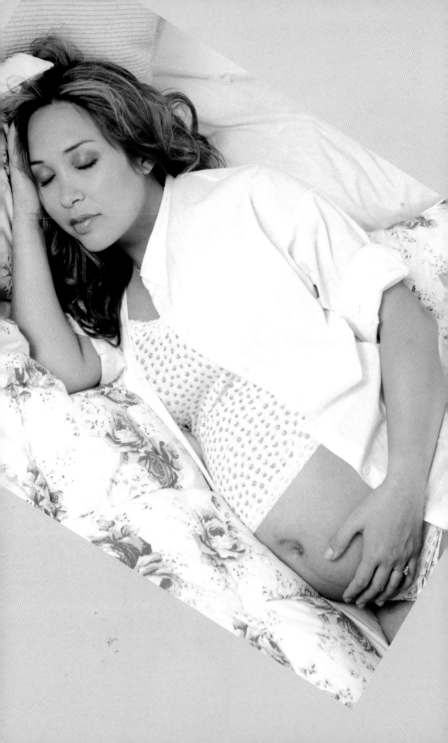

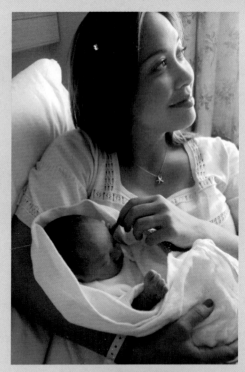

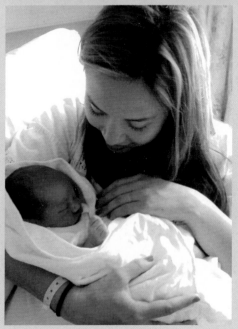

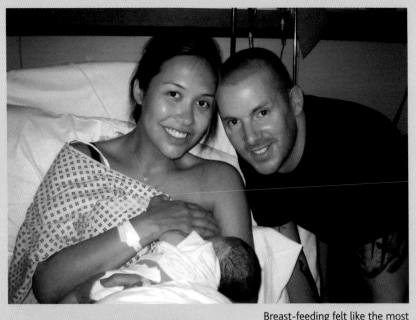

Breast-feeding felt like the most
natural thing in the world.

Nana Ita and Grampa
Willy with their new
granddaughter.

Lola Bong and Grampa Oscar.

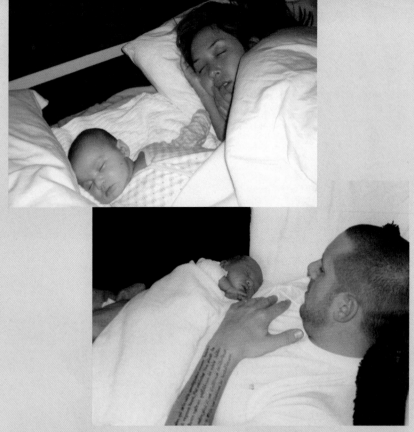

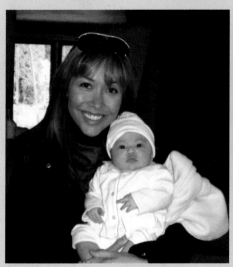

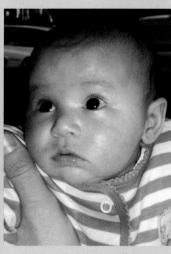

Ava at four weeks.

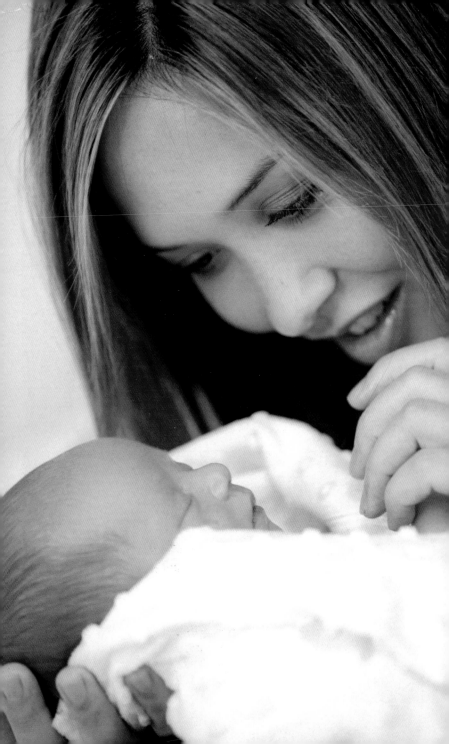

Week 27

The Week We Upset a Monkey in Mauritius

The seat-belt signs were on, the plane was about to land, the pilot did his 'bing bong, welcome to Mauritius' and it was at that moment that I puked up all over Gray and me.

It wasn't the best start to our much-needed holiday. The holiday that – we kept reminding ourselves – would be our last relaxing break for some years.

Being sick was the worst bit of our long journey towards paradise. Gray had decided to surprise me with the trip to Mauritius – knowing that we would be cut off from everything and with no choice but to relax.

Because it is such a long journey we had to have a stopover in Dubai, which was horrendous. When we touched down it was forty degrees, I was desperate for the toilet and getting hot flushes. I was in such a rush to get to the loo that I left my bag behind at the security point and we had a frantic search to find it.

By the time we got on the plane to Mauritius I was absolutely exhausted and managed to sleep through dinner and breakfast. I only woke up fifteen minutes before landing to find I was both desperate for the toilet and starving hungry.

The air steward tried to stop me going to the toilet, telling me the seat-belt sign was on. But with an extremely determined/

My tip Whatever you do, however busy your life is, make sure you take a small break before your baby is born. You will really, REALLY appreciate it once your little whirlwind has entered your life. Holidays really will never be the orgy of relaxation that they once were. Savour the time when it is just the two of you – you might need some happy memories when sleep exhaustion is leading you to snap at each other.

desperate look on my face I told him, 'I am six months pregnant and I need to go to the toilet NOW.' He let me pass.

He refused to find me any food, however, so I managed to rummage up two apples which were at the bottom of my bag. But they must have mixed badly with my empty tummy because as the plane's landing gear came down and the pilot told us we were now in sunny Mauritius that all-too-familiar feeling came over me.

I just about had time to say to Gray, 'I'm gonna be sick,' when I was, all over him.

Luckily we both had blankets and managed to soak up most of the mess. But that wasn't the end of poor Gray's troubles. When we left the airport and found a taxi I promptly fell fast asleep once again on Gray. He suffers from travel-sickness when he sits in the back but didn't want to move because it would wake me up. Bless!

Once we got to our gorgeous hotel, thankfully, it was a different story. Complete and utter bliss and relaxation. We both slept for hours and hours. We relaxed, we ate well and the best thing was we spent time together.

It made me realise how busy things had been since I had come out of the jungle – we were often like two ships that passed in the night. And spending this time with Gray made me realise all over again how much I loved him.

We would talk constantly about Rice, about how next time we went on holiday she would be with us. We would look at families and talk about how that would be us in a few months and we made friends with two other pregnant couples.

We would talk about which countries we wanted to take Rice to, how we wanted her to experience different cultures and how we wanted to bring her back to Mauritius.

Our days took on a slow routine where we would wake late for breakfast, the staff would give me an extra bowl of fruit after spotting me nicking some for later in the day, we would go back to bed, do some sunbathing and then often back to bed before dinner and a movie.

Normally a sun worshipper, the weather was perfect for me now as it was the monsoon season so often quite hazy and not too hot.

I had worried about what effect sunbathing might have on my baby. It's another area of contradiction, with some people saying you should go out in the sun for vitamin D and others saying to avoid sunbathing because of a risk of overheating.

My big worry was that I might blind Rice if she looked up into the sun while I had my belly out.

Dr Mason told me not to fret about that, but warned me to put factor 50 on my face and a high factor on the rest of my body. Pregnant women are much more likely to get sunburned than before because of those pesky hormones making the skin more sensitive. And you will also be prone to skin pigmentation called chloasma. This causes dark patches on your face known by the rather scary moniker of the 'mask of pregnancy'.

That was enough to frighten me into putting on the highest factor I could find.

He also warned me not to get too hot as you can get dehydrated and overheated – so I made sure that I always had a bottle of water and a glass of orange juice near me. And if it did get too hot, unlike the days of old when I would have roasted myself in the sun, I went into the shade.

I had a wonderful time reading books and magazines while Gray – who has never been one to sit down – would go for a run or look for interesting shells on the beach.

Going in the sea was lovely as I felt so light and Gray could even pick me up. But when I would get out I realised how heavy I was. My boobs, in particular, felt like they weighed a tonne and I was getting a bit of neck ache from my halterneck bikinis which were holding them in.

One day it rained so we used the opportunity to go exploring a nearby park and waterfall. Gray had packed a rucksack with enough things to look after a whole army – or a pregnant woman. These included towels, maps, jumpers, sunscreen, phones, local emergency numbers, biscuits, torches and – just for me – some toilet paper.

We went for a hike up to the waterfall and it wasn't long before I needed to use the toilet paper and went behind a tree.

I then heard Gray shouting, 'Leenie, quick, move away from there.' He had a really serious look on his face and added, 'There's a monkey above you in the tree.' I could hear a rustling noise above me but was convinced he was joking and said, 'Pull the other one.'

But he still had the worried look on his face and he was bending down really slowly to pick up a stick. 'Leenie, will you move, quickly,' he said.

And then I looked up and saw this really cute little monkey and it was bouncing down towards me. But as it came closer I could see that it wasn't so sweet – it was swishing its tail and baring its fangs.

It had obviously seen me doing my thing with my big white bottom in the air and had taken it as someone invading his territory.

I tried to run but all I could do was waddle. I finally reached Gray and we backed off as we saw this whole family of monkeys jumping down from the tree and snarling and weeing everywhere – obviously marking their territory back. We made a run for it.

Like all holidays, ours seemed to go both slowly and yet too quickly and before we knew it, it was our last night.

There were tears at our last dinner when Gray turned to me and told me I was the best thing that had happened to him, how we would make a brilliant family and how there was nothing he wouldn't do for his girls.

I immediately burst into tears and couldn't stop. People started giving Gray evil looks as they saw him as the mean man who had upset the poor pregnant lady. He was so embarrassed. I tried to make myself smile so that people could see there was nothing wrong but I couldn't stop crying.

And then we were on our way home. Before boarding our flight from Dubai to London I got stopped at the gate by a man who insisted on seeing my 'fit to fly' letter. I told him that I wasn't 28 weeks yet so didn't need it. The row went back and forth while the queue, which included England footballer John Terry, built.

Eventually he let me on, saying: 'If one of the stewardesses doesn't want you to stay you are going to have to get off.' I quickly grabbed Gray's jumper, which I put on, and wrapped my pashmina around me so they wouldn't notice me.

I got a 'bad seat' next to a woman and her crying baby. In the past I would always have been annoyed but this time I felt so sorry for the poor mother as she couldn't calm her baby down and it looked so distressing.

I knew it wouldn't be long before I would be in the same boat, and watching her try to get her baby to stop crying I was both sympathetic and nervous at the prospect.

What's happening to your body – Week 27

You: Are now at the end of the second trimester and you may already find things are becoming a little harder than they were in the rosy-cheeked glow of the start of this trimester. Extra pressure on your system and water retention could already start causing varicose veins and swelling of the ankles, known as oedema. If you are suffering really badly from swollen ankles you can buy support stockings, which need to be put on before getting out of bed in the morning. Other ways of combating it are to try and put your feet up as often as you can, doing some light exercise like walking and putting your feet in a bowl of cold water.

Your baby: Now measures around 30cm from head to rump – a bit bigger than a sheet of A4 paper – and weighs close to two pounds – just over a quarter of its final body weight. Over the next few weeks of your pregnancy its fat layers will form and it will rapidly put on weight. Your baby can now open and close its eyes, which will be blue if you are white-skinned or brown if you are from an Asian or black background. Your baby's eyes will often change colour in the first six months of its life.

12 June 2007
Gray's Diary

Mauritius 9 a.m.: wake-up call. Been asleep eight hours or more but we still feel knackered. I think the last few months are catching up on Leenie. She feels so tired. I drag her to breakfast because I know she needs to eat. She is still asleep walking around breakfast. She keeps talking to the staff, thinking it's me behind her. Very weird. And I find myself finishing every sentence for her, she just can't get the right words out. These are changes I have noticed over the past few months. Leenie was always very clever and quick thinking but since the baby I find I have to help her out much more. After breakfast back to bed for three hours. Wake her up. First thing's a wee, followed by the words, 'I'm hungry, get me food.' So four bananas, some slices of cake and then finally slap factor 50 on her face, all over bump and boobs and we're ready to go. But only after another wee, of course.

Week 28

The Week There Were Tears Over a Changing Table

There were just three months to go until Rice was due and I knew that she would now have a good chance of survival if she was born. So it seemed like a good time to go shopping.

I didn't have a house to nest in and I didn't even know where we were going to be living when she was born. But I was still determined to have everything ready for my baby.

At first I wanted everything to be pink. I remembered how I loved pink when I was a little girl and I wanted her to have the perfect room. But Gray immediately vetoed that, saying it would just look tacky in our new house and that if she wanted it pink when she grew up then we would change it then.

We eventually agreed to go for neutral colours – although Gray did cave in to my pleas to have star-shaped lights on her ceiling and a princess and fairy mural in our new house.

The first thing we felt we needed was some nursery furniture. But, as I was to discover, even buying the furniture could be an emotional business.

The set we chose had a changing table that matched the cot and the wardrobe and I immediately said, 'That's the one.'

Gray replied: 'No way.' He said that it was up in the air and she could easily roll off. That thought hadn't even occurred to me –

and I was shocked and tearful that I wasn't thinking that way. How could I be a good mummy if I wasn't thinking about the risks? What if we had bought it and she had rolled off and hurt herself?

In a way it was tears for the sake of tears, but I guess I was getting a little bit apprehensive.

Although I couldn't wait to meet Rice, to give her cuddles and see who she looked like, in other ways I felt like I was on the train tracks with a speeding train approaching. I wanted to slow things down, revel in my pregnancy and get everything organised. I didn't feel like I knew enough about being a mummy and I wasn't sure I was ready. There also seemed so much to do and so little time to do it in.

I then discovered that the Mamas and Papas set that we liked wasn't in stock at the store, and that stressed me out as well as I suddenly thought – what if she comes now?

That afternoon we went online to order it and the company said they would do their best to get it to us on time but there was an eight-week wait. And then the PR department got in touch and – incredibly generously – decided to give it to us. You might hear some celebrities moan about fame but I have to tell you it's not all bad!

We also had prams coming out of our ears.

I had become somewhat obsessed by them. I nearly turned into an owl as every time I saw someone walk past me with a pram my head would spin around 180 degrees. I used to be like that with shoes but now I would nudge Gray and say, 'Check out the pram.'

I would watch people at airports to see how they folded their prams and look at them getting in and out of cars to see which was the best travel system. I noticed that some colours were better than others at hiding the mess babies make and I tested out which ones were heavy and which weren't.

And then I was invited by Silver Cross to choose one of their prams and all my research went out of the window. I fell in love with one of their large traditional prams which looked like it had come straight out of Mary Poppins. It didn't fold, was totally impractical and you almost needed a heavy goods licence to steer it, but it was utterly beautiful.

Gray refused to allow me to get it – he said it wouldn't fit into our flat, let alone a shop doorway. And he also quite rightly pointed out that if I got stranded in the rain he would have to hire a van to come and get me.

But I secretly ordered it anyway. Sometimes a mother's just gotta do what she wants to do!

Thankfully for us, we had lots of kind offers from people to give us prams. Mothercare gave our favourite travel system (we particularly loved the name Quinny) and we had more than enough pushchairs to go round. It meant we had more than enough to go around – one for my car, one for Gray's, one for my parents and the Silver Cross which only fitted in the flat.

We were still being offered even more prams so I gave a couple away to my friends and the shelter and then I turned the rest down. Even I could see that a girl can have too many prams.

After the pram came all the rest of the baby paraphernalia. Who would have thought that such a little thing would need SO much stuff?

All the books had lists and lists of things you needed and my friends also gave me their personal recommendations. There was so much information that it was enough to make my head spin. My friends would talk about cellular blankets and muslins and I had no idea what they meant (in fact, for a long time I thought the blankets were called circular blankets).

We ended up with about twenty types of feeding bottles in all shapes and sizes because everyone we talked to had a different one they recommended. And then we would buy one and discover it didn't come with a teat or it didn't fit into the steriliser we had bought. There was so much choice, it was a whole different world.

We also bought lots of things which never left their packets – we had bottle warmers we never used after friends advised us to get her used to drinking the milk at room temperature to save time.

We discovered what a huge industry the baby machine is – and how you can feel pressure to buy something when you don't really need it.

Even the scores of gorgeous pink clothes we had bought or been given for Rice were to remain unused.

What's happening to your body – Week 28

You: Are on the home stretch. You will find the final trimester both goes too fast as you start to panic about how you are going to cope with a newborn and also too slowly as you struggle with a growing bump and get excited about meeting your baby. This week you may have a blood test to check for anaemia, a deficiency of red blood cells, which is common at this time. If your blood group is Rh negative you will have further tests.

Your baby: Is now 34cm, the height of a 1.5l bottle of water, and is getting fatter by the day. Some experts believe that babies begin to dream this week as there is more brain activity, even during sleep – although no one knows what is on their mind.

$\mathcal{M}y\ tip$ There are no hard-and-fast rules about what you really need when you are having a baby but here is my list of essentials for both you and the baby once you have given birth.

For baby:

- **Babygrows** – these are an absolute must and you should have at least eight as you will be staggered how many you will need to wash in a day; it is also a good idea to get at least one pack of tiny baby ones just in case you deliver early

- **Vests**

- **A Moses basket or cot** plus lots and lots of sheets (if you are getting a Moses basket or crib you don't actually need to buy your cot for a few months)

- **Cellular blankets** to wrap baby in

- At least a dozen **muslins and bibs** – the best things in the baby world

- **Steriliser** – go for one that looks easy to use and, if you have time, practise using it before you go into labour, as following instructions is the last thing you will be able to do once you are sleep-deprived

- **Bottles** – get a few small ones to start off with and make sure you get a newborn teat (yup, it's a whole new world – bottle teats come in different sizes for different ages); we chose

Avent bottles mainly because the make is everywhere, so easy to get hold of in case of emergencies

- **Car seat** – again practise putting it in and out of your car and make sure it is ready in your car for the big arrival
- **Nappies** – note that some makes have different newborn sizes according to weight (as if you are not confused enough in those first few days!); get a selection – you can always exchange them
- **Cotton wool** for changing nappies
- **Baby wipes**
- If you are going to bottle-feed choose **a formula** and get some stock
- If you have any intentions of breast-feeding get **a breast pump** – electric ones are easiest to use
- **Nightlights** so that you can reach the baby in the dead of night without tripping up
- **Room thermometer** so you don't have to worry about baby overheating
- **Little bath** which can go inside the big bath – we chose a great one from Mothercare after realising she was a slippery little fish in the big bath
- **Changing mat** – or maybe two in case one gets covered in poo and you need to make an emergency nappy change (get one with a removable towel so it is not too cold)

- **Pram** – look around and see which ones you like being pushed about
- **Papoose or baby sling** – this isn't a must but we both get lots of use out of it and it is a particularly great way to get your partner to feel close to the baby

For you:

- A bumper pack of big **sanitary towels** for when you bleed after the labour – and some **giant knickers** to accommodate them
- **Waterproof sheet** for under your covers in case of a lot of bleeding
- **Breast pads**
- **Snuggly clothes** with big arms to cuddle you in the first shocking few days of motherhood

You will also discover a new appreciation for your WASHING MACHINE, if you have one, as it will become the most used item in your house for several years to come.

Week 29

The Week Questions Started Being Asked About Whether I Should Stop Work

'Is Myleene working too hard?' the magazine asked in its headline. It was a question more and more people were putting to me.

Since coming out of the jungle I had found that I was much more in demand than I had been for years. Instead of putting people off, my pregnancy seemed to attract jobs.

I worked at CNN for six days a month doing their movie show *The Screening Room*, I had a Classic FM radio show twice a week and a Capital FM Sunday-night programme. I was an ambassador for classical music at EMI, contracted to bring out six albums over two years. I also wrote interviews for *Classic FM* magazine. I had a nightly BBC1 evening show, The One Show. And last, but by no means least, I was a model for M&S.

It meant my days were full and I was often working seven days a week. And people – especially other women – began to pressurise me to stop.

Even close friends would try and convince me to put my feet up. 'I stopped at six months . . . I stopped at thirty-two weeks . . . I took four weeks off,' their comments would always be prefaced by, almost like I was judging them by not stopping when they did.

> *My tip* Don't let anyone pressure you into making decisions about when to give up work. You have to do it when you feel you need to. If you are employed, when you tell your employer that you are pregnant you also have to tell them when you intend to start your maternity – this cannot be more than eleven weeks before your due date. If you want to change the date you need to give 28 days' notice unless it is related to illness.

People would say I needed to rest and relax for the baby's sake while some strangers even said it was disgusting to see a pregnant woman presenting on television.

My working obviously polarised opinion. Other viewers would write in and say, 'Good on you, it's great to see a pregnant woman working.' And I got lots of support from other pregnant women saying I was a role model for them, as did some of my friends who had also worked until late in their pregnancy.

Like so many things in pregnancy, when it comes to when to stop work I believe that you have to go with what is right for you.

And I was determined to carry on for a myriad of reasons.

The first, and most important, is that I genuinely love my job. I am not stuck in an office every day bored out of my mind or run off my feet working day and night like nurses. I was travelling, I was meeting interesting people, I was making music and talking music, I was doing something different every day.

When I had days off I was bored. I am a very active person and lying on the sofa watching daytime telly with a calendar and magic marker pen are not my idea of fun.

I had no house to 'nest' – so there was little I could do to prepare for the baby outside of buying the essentials.

I also felt like I had a responsibility to other pregnant women to show that you can do it – pregnancy is not an illness. All those emails that said it was 'unacceptable' spurred me on. This is what happens to women, they get pregnant and they carry on working. I was proud to be a working pregnant woman and I was also determined to be a proud working mother.

And although my work schedule looked ridiculous – and sometimes it was – normally it was workable and not as bad as it appeared. Once I started on *The One Show* my working day would normally start at 2 p.m. when a car came to pick me up and I would be home by eight.

The radio shows only lasted for five hours a week and the M&S shoots were sporadic.

And after the admittedly very difficult first trimester when everything was still a secret (which practically everyone goes through), if I felt things were getting too heavy, I would ask for my schedule to be eased off.

People were very understanding and if I needed to have twenty minutes' sleep in my dressing room, I could. If I thought something would wear me out I would ask for it to be changed. I was sensible – although my work was important to me, my baby always came first.

I am not saying, though, that working through pregnancy is a walk in the park, and I can totally understand why lots of women give up early. I have already described the horrible frustration I felt at my brain disappearing.

It could also be hard being 'a model' or trying to look glamorous on television when all I felt was fat and bloated. And sometimes I would come home so tired I couldn't speak. But I don't think that I was different from any other pregnant woman who works.

One of the weirdest things was trying to explain to people who had no idea about pregnancy why I was behaving like I was. I think you can only really understand baby brain, erratic hormones and growing boobs if you or your partner has experienced them.

This became clear when I had a weird conference with my manager, who is a bachelor, and several of my employers, when we tried to pencil in some time off for me.

After telling Jonathan my 7 September due date could only be an estimate he asked: 'Well, when do you think the baby will come?' I replied, 'Er, I don't know.'

'Well, will it be early?'

'Er, I don't know.'

'If it's early or late what are we looking at here? One week, two weeks?'

'Er, I don't know.'

I was getting hot, frustrated and embarrassed, and surprised that no one around the table understood why I couldn't know exactly when my baby was going to arrive.

The other thing that really spurred me on to keep working was the knowledge that I had to take the jobs while I could. I don't take any job for granted – I have had times there when the phone doesn't ring and the work dries up.

I know that one day my work will stop and I won't just be able to go out and get a part-time job. I take every day as my last, and following my success on *I'm A Celebrity* I knew that I could be enjoying my peak year – even if I was pregnant.

Both Gray and I came from normal families where money could often be tight. It's something that stays with you – and I didn't want that for Rice. Although I also didn't want her to be spoiled, I wanted her to have a nice home, a good education and everything she needed. And these things have to be paid for.

Having said all that, my intention had been to take two weeks off before my due date. I had a box set of Lost I wanted to get through and Gray also finished work early so we could spend some time getting ready.

Little was I to know, however, that Rice had her own plans – and I would be working live on air when she decided she wanted to come out.

What's happening to your body – Week 29

You: If you are planning to do an antenatal class it should start in the next few weeks. You will learn about labour, practising positions with your partner, and also about postnatal care. It will also give you the opportunity to make friends with women in your local area having babies – something that can be a lifeline in the months ahead. It may also be worth you going on a tour of your hospital so you are familiar with the birth unit.

Your baby: Measures 36cm – the diameter of a wok – and weighs 3½lb. It is becoming brainier as both head and brain grow rapidly. It also has fingernails, eyebrows and eyelashes.

Week 30

The Week I Realised I Had Become a Baby Bore

I admit with horror that I used to wonder about what stay-at-home mums could have to talk about, other than babies.

As a workaholic who had an exciting job and loved current affairs I was always convinced that baby talk wasn't something that would thrill and excite me. I also never saw myself as the motherly type and even worried about whether my maternal instinct – which some girls seem to have from the age of ten – would ever kick in.

But when I fell pregnant everything changed. I could talk childbirth, bottles, breast-feeding, nappies and cellular blankets until the cows came home.

I realised exactly how much of a baby bore I had become when Gray and I had our neighbours Mel and Dom for dinner and we talked nothing but babies for three and a half hours.

When you are pregnant even though the world may be at war, there may be a new prime minister and your favourite pop star may be having a public breakdown there really is no subject more fascinating than babies – particularly your own.

I would find anyone that I could to talk babies with. Having noticed that friends without children would only be feigning an interest after an hour or two, I would seek out parents, thinking that at least with them I could indulge in my obsession for another sixty minutes.

I would go to baby shops and buy just one more outfit or giggle and marvel at the clothes as I lay them across my bump. I have already explained how I would prowl the streets looking at prams. And, of course, I also had a peep in to look at the babies inside.

I would spend hours deciding what outfit to put Rice in when we left the hospital. I developed a new love for the colour pink. I would pore over my scan pictures to make out her every little feature.

Everyone I knew with children was bombarded with questions. I wanted to compare how people had done things and how they coped.

Gray couldn't believe the change in me – even though he was as excited as I was. 'What happened to the girl who was all work, work, work?' he used to ask. But I couldn't fight it – I simply didn't want to talk about anything else.

I felt like I had joined this amazing new 'mothers' club'. When I would walk down the street other pregnant women or mothers would give me a smile or a wink, like we had an unspoken understanding.

When my girlfriends had been pregnant themselves I had, of course, been genuinely thrilled for them. But I didn't realise quite what they had been going through.

Now I was having a baby I wanted to shout it from the rooftops and gabble about it incessantly. I was totally obsessed with my pregnancy. I also realised how things would be once I was a mummy proper – when you have to listen to stories of other people's children before you can talk about your own. It's good manners to look at everyone else's pictures but really you are doing it so you can pull out your own photos (even if they are only scans) to show them off.

My tip At first I did really worry about what had become of the strong, hard-working Myleene of old. Then I realised that there was nothing I could do about my baby preoccupation – all I could do was go with it. I found the people who didn't get quite so bored with my obsession were other mothers, my own mother and – obviously – Gray. I also found that writing my diary helped – it meant I could detail every little change in my body without having to explain why I thought it so interesting!

I kept my scan photo on my phone and would bring it out at every given opportunity. Even when I could tell that people's eyes had glazed over and they weren't that interested I would pursue it – I didn't care!

It was incredible, in particular, to talk to other mums-to-be in the same position as me. I was more than lucky that I had Lauren to share everything with. And when I bumped into pregnant celebrities like Charlotte Church we would stand in a corner and talk babies.

Although I hadn't met Rice yet I was already feeling like a mother. And the slightest thing about being a mother would set me off. Stories about the deaths of children would have me in paroxysms of tears. But so would adverts (there was a particular one for Clover in which people were crying over their buttered corn on the cobs which had me in floods).

Then there was the National Geographic channel. When we were watching a programme about a gorilla mother who had rejected her child Gray's mother called in the middle of it and I was so upset that I couldn't even speak to her. I had to hand the phone to Gray.

My obsession about babies wasn't restricted to my waking hours.

As for many women, my dreams became really vivid during my pregnancy. I often woke up thinking they were real. And it doesn't take more than an armchair psychiatrist to work out I was obviously worried about what sort of mother I would be and how Gray and I would cope with parenthood.

One really frightening nightmare came soon after a friend told me that she could recognise her baby's cry in a room of a dozen other children.

I dreamed that I was in a room with lots of babies and they were all crying and I was running around trying to work out which baby was mine and I couldn't tell.

There was another dream in which I had left my baby on the sofa but couldn't find her. I also had nightmares about car accidents and plane crashes, often just before flying. A recurrent dream was that Gray was going to leave me, even though I have always felt 100 per cent secure in our relationship.

I would wake up in a cold sweat thinking we had just had a

What's happening to your body – Week 30

You: Are expected to gain just over one pound a week this trimester as your baby's demand for nutrients is at its greatest. Try and make sure your diet is well balanced with foods rich in protein, vitamin C, folic acid, iron and calcium.

Your baby: Is now 37.5cm long from crown to rump, the height of a bathroom cabinet mirror. Its length growth is slowing down but it is filling out and now weighs over three pounds. Your baby can now probably see its surroundings.

huge argument and he had decided to go. I would even say to him, 'Are we OK?' and he would look at me like I was mad and reply, 'Of course we are.'

Some of my dreams were just plain old bizarre. There was one in which Sharon Osbourne asked me to paint her gargoyle purple. I have no idea where that came from.

And there was another where we had a cat in the fridge. Every time I wanted to get something out of it I had to manoeuvre past it. When I woke up I asked Gray, 'Why is there a cat in the fridge?' He just laughed and said, 'You're nuts.'

Doctors believe the vivid dreams in pregnancy are caused by a combination of hormones, anxiety about what is coming and increasing difficulties in sleeping. And as I approached the final few weeks of my pregnancy I was beginning to experience all three by the truckload.

3 July 2007
Gray's Diary

Tonight I put my face to Leenie's bump to have my talk with Rice, then I started to push the bump with my hands. Then Rice kicked out – she's so strong she kicked my nose. I couldn't believe it, she managed to push my nose. This was the best feeling ever. I can't believe she is that strong and was able to do that to me. For months she was just this little grain growing inside her mama. Now, for the first time, I know that she is nearly ready to come into the world and she is real. This makes me even more impatient and want to see her now. Hurry up, Rice!

Week 31

The Week I Looked Like I Had Been in a Slasher Movie

As I stepped out of the shower I glanced at myself in the mirror. There was blood all over my face, all over my body and now it was all over the floor. I looked like an extra from a horror film.

Fortunately, it appeared more frightening than it actually was. The blood was down to yet another nosebleed. They had started coming in the last few weeks and now I was getting them all the time, particularly after showers.

After hitting the third trimester the wonderful honeymoon period of the last couple of months had ended with a bump as I seemed to be struggling with new pregnancy difficulties every day.

As well as showers, my nosebleeds seemed to be brought on by eating, travelling and heat. I once turned up for an interview for Sky News with two tissues stuffed up my nose as I couldn't get my bleeding to stop.

And as I was just about to film my part for the Marks and Spencer advert in Venice when I was eight and a half months pregnant – fully made-up, in beautiful clothes, with dozens of people waiting for me – another nosebleed decided to make an appearance.

It wasn't the only place I was bleeding from: I would also have lashings of it dripping from my mouth whenever I brushed my teeth,

> *My tip* Always carry plenty of tissues in case of nosebleeds, have lots of water with you to stop dehydration and, if you are feeling really hot, I always found running my wrists under cold water could help. Also, those bouncy balls are fabulous. As well as helping relieve your ribs, they can help engage the baby's head and you can even lean on them during labour. You can get them in many sports shops and your hospital may be able to advise you where else you can get them.

thanks to my newly super-sensitive gums. I can only thank my lucky stars, however, that I didn't ever get the dreaded haemorrhoids – particularly as I was carrying so much extra weight.

From having the small tidy bump of my second trimester I was now just big. People would look at me and say, 'Ooooh, you're gonna have a ten-pounder.' I am not sure what sort of reaction they expected from that – certainly not one of calm.

If I tried to sit on Gray's lap he would not-so-gently remove me, saying, 'I don't want you to break my legs.'

My thighs had got so big that they started rubbing together. And when it was hot a sort of friction rash would appear. I would walk along like John Wayne, not because the baby had dropped but because I had to try and keep my legs apart as the rubbing was so painful.

We did discover an ingenious solution for that particular problem. When I came home in agony one evening and showed Gray he got me to try a stick of cream he used for marathon running. It actually worked a treat.

There were, however, plenty more indignities.

As we lived on the Thames there were plenty of whale jokes from the ever-so-sensitive father-to-be. When it became harder and harder to manoeuvre myself off the sofa and bed and out of the car we perfected what we called 'the whale roll'. Gray would give me a gentle push or pull and I would roll onto my side and then onto my hands and knees.

I began to feel slow and heavy and cumbersome, like I was moving underwater. If I was late for something and tried to hurry up I found I couldn't – I would just get out of breath.

Breathing itself became increasingly difficult as Rice grew even bigger. My ribs began to really ache as my uterus began pushing against it from the inside. I felt like I was constantly bruised and constricted and that the baby was pushing up to my chin. It became difficult to take in full breaths and sleeping was almost impossible – Gray would have to prop me up on lots of pillows.

I did find that sitting on one of those large bouncy exercise balls helped a bit. I would eat my dinner on it and watch TV. I would also spend hours bouncing up and down on the ball, relieved at the way it seemed to take the pressure off my ribs.

Rice's growth also caused a return of my nausea along with a new symptom of acid reflux, which gave me terrible heartburn every time I bent over or lay down. At least by now I knew how to cope with the nausea – and upped my food intake to having something every hour in an effort to combat the feeling of sickness.

I was also in pain in my lower back, thanks to the effort of carrying an extra three stone (and counting). My sister gave me a lavender heat pack, which was wonderful until I realised that it was also giving me hay fever. I would wake up with my back feeling great but my eyes streaming.

I found that often the best cure for all my aches and pains was lying in the bath – I could be in there for hours.

Being in the bath also meant that I wasn't sweating – one of my most annoying symptoms. I felt hot and sweaty and wet all the time and it wasn't even a good summer. I was horrified at the idea of having sweat patches on my clothes so developed an almost nervous tic where I would be constantly checking my underarms. I was also really worried that I smelled.

I would drive Gray mad by constantly questioning him about whether I looked sweaty, whether I needed more deodorant, whether he could smell me. I was really conscious of the sweatiness and felt so much hotter than before.

It is a fact that a pregnant woman's core temperature is higher than normal because of her hormones, increased blood flow and heat produced by the placenta, and I really felt it.

I was lucky that it was one of the worst summers in memory, but while everyone else was wrapped up in cardigans and trousers I would still be dressed for holiday. Sometimes I would stand in front of my fridge or freezer I was so in need of being cool, or I would run cold cans of coke over my head and neck and chest.

Although I was lucky to escape having swollen ankles, my fingers and arms blew up. It was a sad day when I had to take off my engagement ring, although I was also excited as I knew that it was a sign I was nearly there.

Another new symptom was the leg cramps. The first time I got the searing pain in my calf I screamed so much that Gray thought I had gone into labour. In fact I found cramps so painful they were harder than my labour was for me! I couldn't even manoeuvre around my bump to reach my calf – it was always the right one – so Gray had to lift it in the air for me.

The size of my bump also created all sorts of difficulties that I had never envisaged.

Although I perfected a way of putting socks on by lying on the floor, I could no longer do up laces or buckles. One day on *The One Show* the stylist gave me an amazing pair of pink shoes with buckles for my appearance on the sofa. But after taking my flip-flops off I found that I just couldn't get close enough to my feet to do the buckles up. I could hear the floor manager counting down the minutes until we went live on air and I was contorting my body to try and find a way to do them up. In the end, with just a few seconds to go, the floor manager came and did them up for me. I felt about five years old.

I was also constantly underestimating the size of my bump. One time I went to talk to my friend Severine who works at my management company. As I reached her desk my bump knocked over a vase of flowers, which in turn knocked over a pile of CDs which then, domino effect, knocked over another pile of papers.

At dinner I was constantly spilling food and glasses, while I even managed to catch my bump in a photocopier when I pulled out a paper tray, giving it a really big scratch. Another time I shut the door on it while trying to squeeze into a toilet.

What's happening to your body – Week 31

You: Things will become increasingly difficult for you over the next few weeks as your baby and bump become bigger and heavier. Your uterus pressing against your diaphragm may leave you feeling breathless, back ache can begin (or continue), and sometimes the ligaments supporting the pelvis loosen so much that the joint holding the bones together stops working properly – a painful condition called symphysis pubis dysfunction. But keep your chin up – you are nearly there!

Your baby: Now measures 39cm, the length of a hanger, and things are getting a little squashed in your tummy. You may notice fewer movements as your baby has less room to squirm around.

My bump was so big that Gray used to enjoy eating his breakfast on it. It also became a food magnet. I lost count of the number of times I would leave the house with toothpaste or food on my bump – it just seemed to catch everything. One time I came out of the cinema there was a ring of popcorn around it.

Even piano playing became different now I was pregnant. I couldn't sit that near to the keys so would have to move my stool further away from the piano and then lean forward almost with my bottom in the air. It took extra practice just to perfect the technique.

And as for hugging people – I realised that had to stop after I nearly knocked my ex-soldier muscleman fiancé over! Instead, we perfected a different way of kissing and hugging where I would stand sideways on from him.

Knowing that I had nine weeks to go was scary in many ways. I was worried about whether I could cope with being so big for much longer and I was also concerned about how much bigger it was humanly possible to get.

11 July 2007

Gray's diary

Leenie has had a growth spurt in the last few days. It's hard to hug her as I can't get my arms around her bump. She is so big now and she is so hot all the time. She twists and turns all night finding it hard to get comfortable. I use pillows under her bump to support her and get her to drink less water before bed to try and stop her having to go to the toilet five times a night.

Week 32

The Week I Was Desperate to Get a Glimpse of Rice

From the moment I discovered I was pregnant I had a nagging fear about the health of my baby.

If I hadn't felt a kick for a few hours or one of my symptoms failed to kick in I would start feeling anxious. Even at scans when Rice continuously put her hands in front of her face I would fret about what it meant – about whether something was wrong.

I know from talking to all my mummy friends this worrying is perfectly normal – and is likely to continue for the rest of my child's life – and I usually tried to not let my fears get on top of me, or looked to Gray for reassurance if they did.

And then, as I was reaching the end of my wonderful roller-coaster ride of a pregnancy, something happened to one of my friends which knocked me over sideways.

A close friend of mine, who I had been on lots of adventures with, went for her twelve-week scan only to discover that her baby's brain had not formed properly and it was not going to survive. She had to go through the heartache of having to terminate her pregnancy and, because of NHS waiting times, she was going to have to wait a week to have the operation done. A week when she still had to experience the morning sickness and cravings.

I tried to console her on the telephone with tears running down my face. It was heartbreaking to hear a woman in so much pain. She is someone who is such a strong cookie and nothing can describe the agony she was in.

I didn't know what to say and felt guilty that my pregnancy had gone so well. For weeks we had been talking about all the fun things we would get up to with our babies. It had been so exciting.

To cap it all, my old bandmate Suzanne Shaw had just that morning sent out text messages to all my friends inviting them to the baby shower she and another friend, Jill, had organised for me. And the poor woman who had just lost her baby must have received it.

After speaking to her I spent the night crying. Nothing brings home to you more how miraculous a healthy pregnancy is than knowing someone who has not been so lucky.

Other close friends have suffered from miscarriages in early pregnancy, while another very good pal went through IVF hell for months. You realise that for all the joy you are going through there is someone who is in absolute misery because they are unable to conceive or to sustain a pregnancy.

Some people might think I have had it easy. And in many ways I have. Without even trying, I got pregnant with a beautiful healthy girl.

But I have known heartache in my family. I know that you cannot rely on your pregnancy being successful and your child being healthy. Gray's niece is autistic and we know the difficulties that having a child with such a condition can bring.

After my conversation with my friend I became panicked about seeing Rice. Gray tried to comfort me and told me that getting this upset was no good for our own child.

My tip A big bump is almost like an ostentatious display of your fertility. And if you have a close friend who loses a baby or has trouble conceiving you know that for obvious reasons they may want to stay away from you. All you can do is be there for them, let them know that if they ever want to talk, you want to listen, and make sure that they know you are thinking of them. As for fear and worry, it will stalk your pregnancy, but you have to do your best to try and stay as calm as possible. Getting really worried about your pregnancy will not do either of you any good, but if you are feeling particularly stressed or even depressed talk to your doctor or your midwife.

I was lucky that I actually had a scan booked for the next day so I could at least see that she was OK. When my manager tried to move my scan to another day after a job came up I put my foot down and refused to change the time even by an hour.

It was the best and the worst scan I had ever been to. I had been up all night and was so fearful about what I might see. But when we saw her hair, her kicking legs, her eyes and cheeks and nose that looked like Gray's, there was nothing to match the jubilation that we felt.

A week later we got to see Rice even more clearly as we went for a 4D scan to see what she really looked like. As usual the doctors did all their checks and typically, just as the time came for Rice's photo opportunity, she decided to burrow her face into my pelvis and refused to turn around.

After half an hour of trying to get her to move I left to go to *This Morning* where I was playing the piano on a special show for Fern Britten's fiftieth birthday. I almost gave birth there and then when a glitter cannon went off at the end of the piece – nobody had warned me about the noise and it gave me the fright of my life.

I then rushed back to the hospital to see if we could convince Rice to move for the 4D picture. When I got there we found she had indeed moved but now she had her hands over her face. I drank a Diet Coke to try and get her to move again. When that didn't work, I jumped up and down. Next I downed an espresso

What's happening to your body – Week 32

You: By now it is worth familiarising yourself with what the signs of labour are and what your hospital procedure is. The most common clues are regular painful contractions, lower-back pain and period-like cramps, a blood-tinged mucous discharge (known as 'a show') and broken waters. You don't have to have all of them to mean you are in labour and the presence of some of them doesn't necessarily mean you are in labour. And even if you are in early labour, your hospital may send you away if you turn up too early. Always call your hospital for advice if you think labour may have started.

Your baby: Measures about 40cm – the size of a small baguette – and weighs close to 5lb. It sleeps 90 to 95 per cent of the time but its most active period is normally about 3 a.m. to 5 a.m. – when you are asleep. If it does wake you, consider it practice for the middle-of-the-night feeds you will be doing in a few weeks' time.

(while holding my nose, because the smell made me feel sick) and then the doctor even tilted me backwards on the bed. Rice finally removed one hand from her face but kept the other one in front of it, hiding from us.

After trying for close to an hour I said to Gray and the doctor that I'd had enough – moreover, she'd had enough. I became quite tearful when I thought about what we had put her through and said to Gray, 'All that jumping about – what about her little brain?'

'What about yours?' came the reply. 'She is fine, she is surrounded by water.'

I just appreciated that I had a child who seemed to be alive and well. Getting a perfect snap of her in utero suddenly didn't seem so important.

Week 33

The Week I Got Sick and Tired of 'Breast Is Best' Being Rammed down My Throat

People love to tell you what to do when you are pregnant. And the biggest topic about birth which women are lectured on – you could even say bullied – is breast-feeding. 'Breast is best' is the phrase that everyone likes to bandy around and my family were no exception.

So they were all horrified when I told them I didn't think I was going to breast-feed.

'That's what they're there for,' my brother cried.

'It's the most natural thing in the world,' my dad exclaimed.

'I breast-fed all three of you,' my mother pleaded.

'Breast-feeding is so much better for the child,' Gray's sister said.

Only Gray supported me – whatever decision I wanted to make.

Although I never ruled it out completely I felt and had always felt – long before I fell pregnant – that breast-feeding was just one of those things that wasn't for me. I would see mothers feeding their child and I would feel it was lovely but that I just was not the earth-motherly nurturing type to do it.

I was partly put off by horror stories about cracked nipples and agonising boobs. And I also had plenty of friends who had bottle-fed their babies with no ill results.

I had thought about it a lot. I felt guilty. I was made to feel guilty. And I was made to feel like I would be judged as a bad mother just because I wasn't going to breast-feed. There is a real bully culture around breast-feeding and the worst bit is that it is women against women.

When one of my friends asked a midwife to get her son's bottle after his birth she was practically hissed at. And one evening, while sitting in a reception room after doing a show, I met an inspirational mum who had just had her hip replaced, so bottle-fed her newborn because she needed to take so many strong painkillers. She had been told that if she breast-fed she would not be able to walk for a year or more. There was a female GP also in there and she started telling us both about how much better breast-feeding was and ended by saying, 'Myleene, you really need to read my book. It's about pregnancy for dummies.'

I felt so bad for the poor woman who was still standing there, clearly being judged.

I also felt like I was being judged and it made me question myself. I felt like I must have something missing in me for not wanting to breast-feed. I was worried that maybe it was a sign that I wasn't going to bond with my child. I feared that maybe it meant I wasn't maternal and was going to be a bad mother. It made me feel really isolated.

My tip There is an awful lot of pressure put on women to breast-feed but if you feel it is not right for you, stick to your guns. You are not going to make your baby ill by bottle-feeding, nor will you be a bad mother. You can be made to feel terribly guilty but it is your body and you have to do what you feel comfortable with.

But then I also had plenty of friends who had not breast-fed and their children did not seem to be any the worse for it. They were superb mothers, who bonded with their children, and those children were not unhealthy.

I didn't confide my guilt to anyone except Gray. I didn't want my family to know they were getting to me and I didn't want my non-breast-feeding friends to get the sort of guilty pressure that I was feeling. I think it has to be a very personal decision and I would never preach to any of my pregnant friends on such an emotive subject.

In those last weeks of pregnancy another topic that everyone had an opinion on was tiredness. 'Sleep now . . . get as much sleep as you can,' they all told me.

I was sure they were not lying to me but both Gray and I thought we could handle the sleep deprivation. I have never been someone who needs that much sleep and because of my hectic work schedule I was used to getting only a few hours' sleep a night and having long, long days which could mean working for up to twenty hours. Similarly, the nature of Gray's job also meant that he was used to sleeping in four-hour shifts and working at a hectic pace of life.

I struggled to take on board the idea that I would be so sleep-deprived that I would barely be able to function. When my friend told me that in the week after she had her baby she was so tired she thought she was floating I sympathised with her while secretly thinking that would never be me.

I knew that my friends wouldn't be lying to me – and everyone was saying the same thing. But I think maybe part of me was in denial and part of me was really struggling to get my head around what was about to hit me. I would say 'thanks for the warning' while refusing to buy into it.

The other thing all our new parent friends kept on telling me was that I needed to get some sort of routine in my life for the baby. Some said I should even start getting her into a routine while I was still pregnant. Plenty foisted Gina Ford on me, saying they swore by her Contented Baby series of books in which she sets strict routines for babies.

But I was a free spirit. My own life had totally no routine in it, so I thought there was no way I would be able to get my baby into any sort of routine before she was even here!

I tried reading Gina Ford and it felt far too regimented and extreme. It was like going back to school and having a full curriculum.

I wanted Rice to be a free spirit too and not be issued with her first timetable on arrival. I wanted her to accompany me to work and I wanted her to slot into my life and not the other way around.

It wasn't to be long, though, until I was eating my words. Almost all of them.

What's happening to your body – Week 33

You: Just as the water retention may be making your feet and ankles fill with fluid, it can also swell the nerves of the wrist, causing something called carpal tunnel syndrome, which creates pain, numbness and tingling in your wrists and fingers. There are ways of alleviating it, including wearing a splint or brace, and yoga can also help. If you are feeling very uncomfortable, talk to your doctor.

Your baby: Measures 41cm head to rump, the height of a pillow, and its brain is still developing rapidly. Your baby now has its five senses in place and can see the amniotic fluid around it, feel the sensation of sucking its thumb, taste the amniotic fluid it is drinking and hear your heartbeat and your conversations. There is no air to carry scent in the sac but your baby's sense of smell is already developed and it will be able to smell your milk as soon as it leaves the womb.

Week 34

The Week We Had to Suddenly Move House

We had known for some time that our flat had someone who was interested in buying and wanted to be in quickly.

But we had been so busy with work and getting ready for Rice that we had not thought about the fact that we would soon be exchanging.

And then, suddenly, the sale was going through. We had six days to pack up four years of stuff and find somewhere else to rent, as our new house was far from ready.

I was right in the middle of a really busy period at work and was already totally exhausted. But Gray was my hero, my caveman provider. He set to work finding somewhere to live and quickly found a gorgeous flat right on the Thames a couple of streets from our old home.

And then he started to move us out.

It was an emotional time for both of us. I was in tears as I walked from room to room, thinking about the happy years we had spent there. The idea of being in a new flat where I couldn't nest or even hang up pictures was also a little unsettling – although we both appreciated what a lucky situation we were in. But there were more tears when it came to my wardrobe – this time mainly out of frustration.

Gray told me to just pack what I would need in our new flat as it was smaller than our old one and most of our things would be going into storage. He said I could only fill six boxes of clothes.

But it was impossible to know what I needed. What size would I be? How many maternity clothes should I take? Which shoes would I need? And then there was the whole question of the change in season meaning I would need both summer and winter clothes. It was almost too much!

Even more difficult was the fact that by now I was too big to actually be of any help. Gray forbade me from packing or even carrying my things up and down the ladder to our mezzanine where most of my clothes were stored.

I am used to being a hands-on woman. In the jungle I had even carried stuff for some of the boys (who shall remain nameless!). I felt guilty as I saw Gray pack up our belongings.

My job was to point at what I wanted to be packed and I then had to hide my face in my hands as he and my father threw my

My tip It's a truth universally acknowledged that a couple about to have a baby always leave their house move or redecoration until the last minute. All my friends have done it and I was no exception. If you can organise for the stressful move or building work to happen a little earlier in your pregnancy, then well done you. But if you are like most people and have left it until just a few weeks before the baby's arrival, my only tip is 'don't panic'. Your baby won't notice the chaos around it — all it will care about is that you love it, feed it, clothe it and change its nappy.

gorgeous clothes and shoes down the stairs towards me.

Things became even more slapstick when Gray then dropped his precious fish tank on his foot, making it almost impossible for him to walk.

Goodness knows what our new neighbours must have thought of us when they saw us slowly moving our bits in. We looked like the Trotters, with Gray hobbling along on one foot carrying a sack of potatoes while I was waddling next to him and pushing the Silver Cross pram full of pots and pans.

But I was so proud of Gray for the way he had worked so hard to make the move as painless as possible. He had always said he would look after me and Rice and he'd proven true to his word.

What's happening to your body – Week 34

You: May already have started your maternity leave – some women leave work eleven weeks before their due date, others decide to work right up until the labour. If you do have time on your hands it is a good idea to stock up on wholesome food like casseroles for the freezer to make your life easier once you are coping with a newborn and the accompanying sleep deprivation.

Your baby: Measures 42cm, the length of a casserole dish, and is probably head down in the uterus. If it is in a breech position – with its bottom or feet presenting in the lower part of your uterus – you don't need to worry about it yet; only about 3 or 4 per cent do not turn around by week 37. But there are ways you can help to get it to turn which your doctor or midwife will advise you on.

27 July 2007
Gray's Diary

I got the call to say the sale of our house is going through next week, which only leaves me six days to find a new place to live until our house is finished, move all our stuff out and store some of it. Leenie is going to freak. Oh well, I'm good at fixing things so I know I will make it work. I can do most of it but it's a stressful time. We have so much stuff in this place, it's hard to believe we have managed to fit it all in.

Leenie is working during the days so I can do a lot but I need her help to do all her clothes/bags/shoes etc. and, trust me, this is a six-day job in itself. How can one girl have so much stuff? She must have over a hundred pairs of shoes and even more bags and enough clothes to dress a small country. She doesn't throw anything away so this is going to be a nightmare.

She tells me each night that tomorrow she will do everything. Days pass and we are down to the last two days. I have a go at her to sort it out or they will be going in the bin. My threats work but I'm stressed out. She wants some clothes to go to the new place, some to storage, some to I don't know where! She needs clothes for now, after baby, summer, winter. I'm going off my head.

Week 35

The Week My Friends Showered Me with Love and Pink Things

Looking back on the days before I discovered my inner mama, I feel guilty about my lack of awareness about what all my mummy friends were going through.

It wasn't that I didn't care, or that I didn't bring their children lots of toys or even that I didn't baby-sit for them. On occasion I even cleaned their houses.

But once I became aware of how difficult pregnancy and having a baby are I knew there was so much more I could have done for them. I am so filled with admiration about the way they handled the whirlwind that came into their lives. They managed to cope with family life and work and they still had time to be good friends to me.

The ones who coped with it single-handedly, in particular, still amaze me with their resilience and strength.

My friends seem to have forgiven my shortcomings, however, as they threw me a baby shower to remember.

It was Suzie, a single mum and one of my best friends, who came up with the idea and the party was held at Jill's house. The decoration was pink, pink and more pink.

Mates from where I grew up in Norfolk mixed with friends I had made when I was dancing and singing, people from my management office and my mum. Hardly any of the girls knew each other before the baby shower but all the mummies got their pictures out and there were 'oooohs' and 'ahhhhhs' emanating from every corner.

We talked babies for close to four hours. I was given cellular blankets, muslins, dummies, toys and the most beautiful clothes. I could talk about my pregnancy to my heart's content. There was plenty of drink for the frazzled mothers and single girls, while for Lauren and me there was nonalcoholic wine. I was surrounded by my favourite girls. It was sheer bliss.

I can't shout out enough thanks to all my girlfriends who have been and continue to be my gurus and inspiration. They have made me realise how strong the sisterhood can be and how wonderful female friendship is.

Top of the list has to be Lauren who, with a due date only five weeks after mine, has gone through every step of this journey with me.

My tip Your friends really come into their own when you have a baby as they are the ones who will give you practical and emotional advice that you won't find in books. It is amazing to have them to talk to when you are still pregnant because they can explain things like what a muslin is for. And after the birth they give you help and companionship and reassure you that you are doing OK.

Every fear, every joy has been shared with her. I know I am so lucky to have such a close friend accompanying me at this amazing time. It made the pregnancy for both of us and took the pressure off, as we understood how the other was feeling.

There were often times when even Gray couldn't fathom my behaviour but Lauren could.

And then there are all my mummy friends who are too numerous to mention. There were the ones who were always on hand to offer advice and support. One volunteered to go and get all my bottles, steriliser and all the bits, knowing I might be too busy and tired.

Another offered to shave me 'down there', saying that when she had her baby she'd heard someone else say the doctor had 'plucked me like a chicken' so it was important to keep things tidy, which isn't easy with a bump.

What's happening to your body – Week 35

You: Are probably feeling like a beached whale as your pregnancy uterus – which has expanded to a thousand times its original volume – reaches the bottom of your ribcage. Moving about takes a lot more effort. Try and get as much rest as you can – you are going to need it in the coming weeks.

Your baby: Measures 44cm, about the length from the tips of your fingers to your elbow, and weighs more than 5.3lb. It is getting rounder as it develops layers of fat to help regulate its body temperature.

There were the ones who gave me advice about not putting too much pressure on myself to be the perfect mummy and who were there with a shoulder to cry on during the numerous teary episodes. Others gave me practical advice about what formula I should use or tips like how I should only offer the baby milk at room temperature to save myself from having to warm up bottles.

And it was fantastic to hear that all the other mummies too had experienced everything I was going through: changes in personality, changes in their relationship, changes in the way they saw themselves. It was nice to know that I wasn't the only person to be going through these things.

I have much more in common now with my mummy friends, but my pals without children were just as important. They helped me keep a sense of perspective by talking to me about things other than babies. Even I appreciated the (occasional) change of subject.

Week 36

The Week I Started Panicking About Being a Mummy

'Not long to go now,' Dr Mason beamed at me at our weekly checkup. I am not sure what happened, but a switch flicked on, I turned bright red and my stomach started churning with anxiety.

Aggghhhh! I was going to be a mummy. Responsible for a little person for the rest of her life.

I was scared. Excited and scared.

I'd had nearly nine months to prepare but I still wasn't sure I was ready. I felt like I still had stuff to organise. I am not sure exactly what had to be organised but I just felt that I didn't have everything in place. I thought I needed to read more books. And I wasn't sure that I was properly prepared for the arrival of the little being that was going to change my life. Forever.

At the same time, I wanted her to come now. Everything seemed to be going so slowly and I thought the next few weeks would be the longest I had ever known.

I could see why the gestation period is nine months – Mother Nature (as well as being evil) is awfully clever. I had gone from 'Oh God, I'm pregnant' to 'I'm in hell' to 'This is quite cool now' to 'Come on, it's time now.'

Gray was going up the walls with impatience. Every morning he would wake me up by talking to my tummy saying, 'Come on, Rice, when are you coming?'

And I was desperate to meet her, to see what she looked like, to work out her personality. I was also looking forward to not being huge and heavy any more.

Her crib was set up, her wardrobe was full of clothes, I'd even done a baby first-aid course for emergencies and I had my hospital bag packed.

The only thing left to do was get through the labour.

I had heard a million and one labour horror stories from men and women. It's something that people want to share with poor pregnant girls – and they don't seem to mind frightening you.

From women tearing and 48-hour labours, to heads getting stuck and bloodbaths. I could go on but I know I used to think, 'What have you gained by trying to freak me out with these stories?' No one ever seemed to want to share stories of good labours, yet I know lots of people who have had them.

Despite all the stories, however, I wasn't frightened. I knew that I was going to meet my baby – what could be better than that?

I have been in life-or-death situations – my helicopter was fired on when I went to entertain the troops in Afghanistan, and I also had an unfortunate encounter with a gun in Eygpt. And I knew this was about life.

Lots of books and midwives advise you to have a labour plan but my doctor was against it, being of the view that you can't plan for the unknown.

But I was pretty certain about how I wanted the labour to go. I wanted it to just be me and Gray. I didn't want him down the business end and I wanted an epidural.

Having an epidural is, in some people's minds, a bit like not breast-feeding. There is a lot of pressure on you not to have

$\mathcal{M}y$ tip If you haven't already, it is now time to start packing your hospital bag. Don't do what we did by taking every baby thing you have (see my list below) and also don't do what we did and forget to take pyjamas for you and some essentials for the father (although bear in mind that most hospitals do not allow the father to stay over).

My labour bag contained:

- Babygrows
- Baby vests
- Nappies
- Cotton wool
- Nappy-rash cream
- Hat
- Mittens
- Socks
- Tonnes of clothes for baby (including three dresses), none of which fitted her
- Blankets
- A cardigan
- An electronic thermometer (totally unnecessary thing to take to a hospital)
- Gripe water (ditto)
- A toiletry bag for me
- Big sanitary towels
- Big knickers
- Postnatal bra
- A tracksuit

painkilling drugs, especially from other women who like to tell you about their 24 hours of agony.

I know why women refuse drugs. Having a totally natural birth is a bit like climbing a mountain, a real achievement. But my view was that you don't get a medal for not having pain relief. If you see mothers walking down the street you won't be able to differentiate between the one that had the epidural and the one who didn't. All mothers deserve medals, whether they had pain relief or not.

I'd heard lots of stories of women going through fifteen-hour labours in agony and then deciding they wanted an epidural and not being allowed it because it was too late. I thought, I don't want to be so exhausted that I can't enjoy it and enjoy her.

Instead of being worried about the labour, I was more fearful about what sort of mother I would make. Would I know what to do? Would I make mistakes? Would I do right by her? Would I be good enough?

And I was also desperately concerned about Rice's health. I know I will not be alone when I say that – it's something you can't take for granted.

Despite Gray constantly telling me she was a fighter, she had strong genes, etc. etc., there was a big part of me that thought there is no way of knowing that everything will be OK.

It was another reason why I was looking forward to the birth. I hoped it meant that I could stop worrying.

I didn't realise it would be the start of a whole new worrying experience.

What's happening to your body – Week 36

You: May have developed the 'nesting' bug where you feel you need to prepare your house for your baby by madly cleaning, tidying and ironing. Not so easy when you have a heavy bump, so take care and get help if you need it.

Your baby: Measures approximately 46cm, the height of a footstool, and weighs about 5½lb. Your bump will probably start to 'drop' in the next few days as your baby's head 'engages' into your pelvic cavity. This should help any breathing problems but walking may become a little uncomfortable and you will begin to waddle.

Week 36+6 days

The Day Ava Bailey Quinn Decided She Wanted to Come out While Her Mummy Was on Live Television

I had noticed for a few days that my baby brain had suddenly disappeared and I could remember things again. I joked to friends that maybe this meant the baby was on her way – and it was nature's way of making sure that I didn't lose her.

But I never actually thought I could be right.

August 15th started with a checkup with my doctor, who decided to do an internal to see where Rice's head was. He said everything was lovely and we made an appointment to see each other again in four days' time.

But almost from the moment I left Dr Mason's surgery I started feeling really peculiar. I felt like I had my period coming and was a bit achy around my back and lower abdomen. I didn't think I was in labour, though, I just felt weird.

So I carried on with work as normal, waddling around London with my mini wheelie suitcase I had started taking everywhere with things I would need for the big day.

I went to Classic FM where I did some bits for my radio show. I went to Drury Lane to present some links on the *Lord Of The Rings* musical for CNN. Next I got to *The One Show* studios where I did an interview for British Forces Radio.

Then I sat in make-up, in preparation for the evening's show. I still didn't feel right – in fact I felt even worse and I said to the girls backstage, 'I feel really strange.' Knowing that could often mean I might puke, they went and got me a doughnut.

During the programme, I carried on feeling the ache you get when you have a period but it was becoming more and more painful. I was trying to concentrate on my job and focus on orchestrating live links but at the same time I was wondering what was going on with my body.

I had heard that internals can trigger labour but I thought it more likely that the baby's head had engaged. I didn't twig that I could be in the early stages of labour at all.

After the show we had a bit of discussion about what was happening the following day. We were planning to break a record on the show by getting thirty Elvises in to sing 'Always On My Mind', and I was going to play the piano. As we talked they showed me an Elvis jumpsuit that Adrian was going to wear.

'Let me try it on,' I begged. 'I reckon I'll fit into it, I can be Elvis gone to seed.' I larked about and posed for pictures but then, all of a sudden, I started feeling really bad.

'I need to go home. I need to go home, now,' I said.

I got in the car to take me home and was given the usual labour horror story from the driver about how his wife had endured forty hours of agony before their daughter was born by Caesarean section.

I rang Lauren and said, 'I feel really weird.' She joked that her mum had always said that labour feels like period pains and we were both laughing – never imagining this could actually be it.

Because my mobile phone cuts out in the lift to our flat I sat on the stairs at the bottom of the hallway talking to her for forty minutes until Gray came around the corner and dragged me upstairs.

'I feel really odd,' I told Gray. 'You are odd,' came the reply.

I decided to get in the bath, thinking it might make me feel a bit better. But as I manoeuvred myself in – BANG – the pains got a lot stronger.

'Do you think you might be in labour?' Gray asked.

'I can't be,' I said. 'I haven't had a show, my waters haven't broken. It's not like the movies or what the books say. I just feel a bit weird.'

Before I knew it, two and a half hours had elapsed. I had rolled a towel into a pillow, which I had my head on and was determined to stay there. I looked like someone from Kiss as my mascara was smeared across my face but I couldn't get out – every time I stood up the pain felt a lot worse.

I thought that it must be Braxton Hicks – the practice contractions. I was sure that it wasn't labour and I didn't want to be one of those women who phone up their hospital with practice contractions.

Gray came in and said, 'You can't go to sleep in the bath,' and I said, 'I can. Leave me.'

He started to flick through the books and from what he could tell, I wasn't in labour.

I said to Gray, 'If these are practice contractions, how the hell am I going to get through the labour? This pain is unreal.'

In the end he said, 'That's it, you are going to get out of the bath and we are going to see Mel.' She is our neighbour who also happens to be a nurse.

As I got out of the bath I dropped onto the floor in pain. But then, seconds later, I felt fine.

We both felt a bit fraught and anxious. He kept asking me, 'Are you in labour?' and I would shout back, 'I don't know!'

'Well, do you think you are?'

'I DON'T KNOW!' We seemed to squabble about it for ages. We read through the books together and although they said there might not be a show, and your waters might not break, one said the contractions should be lasting for about a minute. Mine, which were coming every four or five minutes, were only lasting for about twenty seconds.

In my delusional state I also thought I couldn't possibly be in labour because I didn't have my pyjamas.

M&S had just that day sent me some maternity ones but I had missed them at the BBC and was due to pick them up the next day. I know it seems like a weird thought, but it preoccupied me.

We decided to walk to Mel's house, even though by now it was gone 11 p.m., to see if she could shed any light on the matter. As I waddled along I kept on stopping and being doubled over in pain, and then I would be fine.

As we rang the buzzer I had another painful contraction but by the time she opened the door there didn't seem to be anything wrong.

I felt so embarrassed. We had woken up the whole house, including Mel's mother and her baby. And I looked fine.

Mel said, 'Do you think you are in labour?'

I said, 'I don't know.' And the same roundabout conversation I'd had with Gray started all over again. She told me that I might be in early labour but obviously was not about to have the baby straightaway as I could still hold a conversation, and she advised that we call our hospital.

We made our way home and I phoned the hospital. They suggested that we come in to check me out.

Gray grabbed all our bags, even though I thought he was wasting his time.

But as soon as Gray started driving the pain went up by about a hundred notches. It was excruciating.

The only way I could get comfortable was to crouch on the front seat hugging the headrest with my bum in the air. The journey seemed to take forever, and every time we went over one of what seemed like hundreds of bumps, my pain doubled.

When we got to the hospital I slumped down in the doorway in agony. A few seconds later, however, we walked in like there was nothing wrong. I worried that the doctors might think I was making it up.

But a midwife said she would examine me and she discovered that I was two and a half centimetres dilated.

'You are not going home tonight,' she told us.

Gray and I were in shock. 'How long until we see our baby?' we asked. By this time I was crying with excitement.

'You should have her in your arms by four or five o'clock tomorrow afternoon,' came the reply.

And she said that to hurry things along she would do a sweep. This is when they fiddle around with your cervix in order to get it to open more. It is very, very painful.

After she was done she said I could have the epidural I had already requested.

'Now you need to try and rest and conserve your energy.'

I'd heard terror stories about the huge long needle used to administer the epidural but my only trouble with having the injection was that I was giggling so much.

The doctor giving the epidural told me I needed to 'hunch over like a prawn'. That had me in stitches. I think I must have been delirious because I also couldn't stop going on about how I didn't have my pyjamas and the fact that I was supposed to be performing for all the Elvises. I was worried that she might miss my spine because I was shaking so much with laughter. She must have thought I was nuts.

Once the epidural kicked in, it was wonderful. Like magic. The injection felt like ice cubes down my back and then I was no longer in pain. I could still feel a slight pull when I was having a contraction but it didn't hurt at all.

The midwives then pulled out a camper bed for Gray in our room and told us to get to sleep. But we couldn't. Firstly, Gray realised that he hadn't brought any change of clothes for himself for what was likely to be at least a two-day stay. So he rushed home to get a bag of stuff for himself while I thought about what was to come.

Both of us were too excited too sleep. When Gray got back to the hospital we talked for four hours about our past and our future. We were both so excited and nervous knowing that it was the last time when it was just going to be the two of us. We talked about the journey we had been on and how we had to make everything perfect for this baby.

We could sense Rice in the room with us. I was hooked up to a monitor and we could see her heart beating as we talked. We were nearly a little family.

Every time the pain started up again, the doctor would come and top up the epidural and it would disappear. Gray kept on asking to help administer it but I said, 'Please don't listen to him.' The midwives kept on entreating us to go to sleep but all we could think about was that our baby was coming.

Around 5 a.m. we both collapsed with exhaustion, holding hands. I had another sweep at 6 a.m. but I was so knackered that I went straight back to sleep.

$\mathcal{M}y$ tip Next time around I will know
that practice contractions,
while they can be uncomfortable, do not really hurt.
Real ones DO! When it comes to labour, don't be a
martyr. Phone your hospital if you have any worries
and take the drugs if you want them.

By 7 a.m. we were up again when Mr Mason came to check me over. Because my labour was still progressing quite slowly and he thought the amniotic sac might be in the way, he came at me with what looked like a huge knitting needle to break my waters.

By 9 a.m. I was six centimetres dilated and then it just raced. The midwives told me not to eat anything because they didn't want me to be sick during labour – but every time they left the room Gray secretly fed me ice cream.

I barely even felt like I was having contractions. Gray and I were busy making phone calls (I rang Lauren and my family) and putting together lists of all the people we needed to contact to tell them the news.

I could hear a woman in another room screaming with pain from her labour but even when I was 10cm dilated I was on my BlackBerry – that's how magical an epidural is. If I did feel any pain at all I would inhale the gas and air – a rather wonderful drug that makes you feel like you are floating.

At 1.20 p.m. Dr Mason turned up in his scrubs and, although the midwives had told us Rice would probably not be with us until late in the afternoon, I realised that the big moment was about to start – it was time to push.

Just as we were about to get into position, some beef stroganoff that I had ordered turned up.

'You have it, Gray,' Dr Mason said. 'You are going to need the strength to help Myleene push.'

So Gray shovelled it into his mouth and by 1.30 p.m. we were ready.

I was sitting up with one leg on my doctor, one leg on my midwife and Gray holding onto my back.

I thought this process would take hours, but three pushes later and her head was out.

'Do you want to hold her?' the doctor said, guiding my hands to her head and signalling to Gray to do the same. Another two pushes and then, at 1.43 p.m., she was out, into my arms and then straight onto my chest. I looked into her eyes and she looked back at me.

Gray and I were both laughing and crying at the same time. She was here. She was beautiful. Our little baby.

I held her tight and Gray cut the cord. 'Hello, Ava Bailey Quinn,' he said.

After the cord was cut there was a heart-stopping moment when there was absolute silence and then she started squeaking. It was the most beautiful sound I have ever heard. I knew then and there that I was so in love with this little one that I would die for her.

After the labour I was given an injection to expel the placenta and then the midwives wanted to take Ava to get her weighed and checked over. I asked Gray to go with her. And after all the madness I was left all alone. The two people I loved most in the world were in the room next door.

They were only gone for a couple of minutes but it felt like ten hours.

Then the doctor came in to give me two stitches, although I had not torn too much.

Gray and Ava returned – and he announced the baby everyone had told me was huge was a tiny 5lb 9oz – and we spent several minutes all just looking at each other. She was so tiny that she didn't fit into any of the pretty clothes we had brought with us – the only things that didn't totally swamp her were the tiny baby vests that we had.

But she was gorgeous. I thought she looked like Gray while he said she looked like me.

Gray told me how she had already recognised his voice and had stopped crying when he talked to her.

Now she was grizzling again and our first job as parents was to feed Ava.

Gray went with our midwife Sharon to find the formula and they seemed to be gone forever (Gray and I reckon this may have been a deliberate stalling tactic, as she made him fill out loads of forms). When we were alone, just Ava and me, I realised that I needed to feed her. And I wanted to breast-feed her.

I know lots of people have trouble getting their baby to latch on but Ava just did it. She 'rooted' – meaning she turned her head towards my breast as she could smell the milk – and then manoeuvred herself towards it. It felt like the most natural thing in the world.

By the time Gray and Sharon returned, Ava was hungrily feeding. 'Do you need any help?' the midwife asked. But we were fine, instinct had kicked in.

Within an hour and a half our small room was party central as my family and close friends turned up to meet Ava. I was high on adrenaline and a little bit of champagne. I felt like I could run a marathon. I was eating fish and chips and doughnuts and downing

Diet Coke. The flowers started arriving and at one point there must have been twenty visitors crammed into our tiny room. Everyone was so happy for us.

As evening approached I suddenly felt totally exhausted.

But I discovered that I could no longer sleep soundly. Every time Ava stirred or made a little noise from her plastic cot in our room I jumped out of bed to make sure she was OK.

All night I was listening out for her, I wanted to make sure she was all right.

It had been the most incredible day. A fantastically easy labour. A perfect baby girl. But I was about to discover that my difficulties were to come.

What's happening to your body — Week 37

You: Are probably desperate to meet your baby by now – unless you are still at work. If you are at home, listen to your body and rest when you need to. Refresh yourself on information about signs of labour and its different stages. Make sure your car seat is fitted and practise putting the buggy up and down.

Your baby: Is now officially full term and measures about 48cm and weighs approximately 6½lb. All of its organs are developed and it will even have some hair on its head. Because conditions are getting so cramped in the womb don't worry if you don't feel as many kicks as normal – as long as you have a few per day. If you are worried at all about any dramatic change in foetal movement, go and see your doctor.

16 August 2007

Gray's Diary

2 a.m. This is it, the moment I have been waiting for. These months have seemed like years they have gone so slow. I have wanted to be a dad for so long and now it's going to happen. I'm in shock. Don't know how to put it, I have mixed feelings running through my head. One part of me is ready to be a dad, the other thinks, will be I be good at this? Will I do the right things? Will I be able to support my family? And this is the end of my old life; what bits will I miss?

Life has been good to us both and this is going to be the start of another journey. This time we will have a new passenger on board. Even though I'm looking forward to this, a small part of me is scared about what lies ahead.

5 a.m. Leenie's asleep but I'm lying here with a million thoughts running through my head. Typical Catholic — I don't pray that much but tonight I go ahead and ask that everything will be safe and OK.

10 a.m. I have only seen labour in the movies so it is mad to see Leenie being so strong, sitting up and texting people and making lists of people we need to contact.

1.25 p.m. Dr Mason comes in and tells me to eat my dinner quick as Leenie is ready to start pushing. I'm thinking the next few hours I'm going to see her going through the worst pain ever, screaming, calling me every name under the sun. But after three big pushes I can see Rice's head. I'm in shock. I put my hand on the baby's head and tell Leenie to look down, it's an amazing sight. Two more pushes and she comes.

Total silence. Feels like minutes have passed and not a sound from Rice. We are both holding her. And then the moment I will never forget until the day I die, a cry comes from her. Our little Ava has come into the world. I try to cry with happiness but I am past crying and am in a place I have never been.

What's happening to your body – Week 38

You: Take the opportunity to go to the cinema and read some books – you won't get a chance to do them again for some months. It is also worth glancing through a book about looking after your baby – although it might be difficult to get your head around. Try and relax as much as possible as this will seem like a halcyon period in the weeks to come.

Your baby: Measures 50cm – about the size of newborn baby! – and weighs nearly 7lb. Still don't know what you are having? Some clues could be in the way you look. Do you have a big bump? Boys are generally a bit heavier than girls at birth. Some mothers who have girls swear their nose got wider in the last couple of weeks. Girls are also supposed to have faster heartbeats than boys.

My Bump and Me

What's happening to your body – Week 39

You: Yup, you're still waiting. Unfortunately the magic due date that has been circled in red for the last nine and a bit months is unlikely to be the day you actually go into labour. Only 5 per cent of babies are born on their due date and most are later, especially if they are first babies.

Your baby: Measures over 51cm and weighs over 7lb. Its skull is still soft. This means that when it pushes its way through the birth canal its bones will slide over each other, moulding the head into a smaller shape. Once your baby is born its head bones will take about a year to completely join together – at first it will have two soft spots known as fontanelles at the back and on the top of its head.

What's happening to your body – Week 40

You: If you are still waiting you will only have a little bit longer to go. Most doctors will only wait ten to fourteen days after your due date before inducing your baby. If you are feeling desperate there are plenty of old wives' tales about how to make things move a bit faster. These include having sex, eating curries and pineapple, going for walks and having acupuncture. Who knows if they really work – but at least they will keep you occupied.

Your baby: Measures 52cm and weighs over 7½lb. Although most of its organs are ready for the outside world many babies get mild jaundice in the first few days of their life because the liver is not operating fully. It usually settles within a few days but if you are worried at all you should see your doctor.

The Week We Started Our New Life

Twenty-four hours after Ava was born we got the all clear to take her home.

There were about a dozen press photographers outside but I didn't want to expose her to that sort of media scrum when she was still so delicate and precious. I also wanted her to be checked by my midwife before I introduced her to the world.

So – *Goodfellas* style – we left through the kitchen.

But even getting home proved dramatic. We had assembled the car seat according to the instructions but when we put Ava in it and started to drive, her head started flopping about and I was seriously unhappy. We tried tilting the seat and drove so slowly that even bicycles were overtaking us but every time we drove over a bump her head would lollop over.

In the end we stopped the car to see if there was another way of getting the seat in. We hadn't even noticed, but we were right outside the Houses of Parliament on a red route. I was holding Ava while Gray, my brother and sister were all trying to work the car seat out.

All of a sudden a police car turned up behind us. 'Can we help you?' the officers said accusingly.

But when I turned around with Ava in my arms and a pleading look on my face they obviously took pity.

'We heard you'd had a baby, congratulations,' they said, grinning. They were both daddies too – so they also had a go at the car seat to see if they could make it steadier for Ava.

They couldn't work it either – we later discovered it was because we hadn't fitted the newborn cushion onto it – so our journey home was somewhat stressful as I sat in the back trying to hold Ava's head upright.

That evening we phoned the local health clinic to check when the midwife might be coming, as the weekend was coming up and I was extra-anxious to see them because Ava was premature. They assured me that they would either come on Saturday or Monday and I looked forward to meeting someone who could give me advice and check Ava was OK.

And then our nightmare began.

It was the weekend, we had just brought our new baby home and so everyone we knew (and a few we didn't) thought it would be a brilliant idea to come and visit us. People were texting for my new address – I thought they wanted it to send flowers – and then an hour later they would arrive. 'Oh, we were in the area and wanted to meet the baby . . . it's the only day we can see her . . . I just wanted to bring some presents over.'

At first it was fine as Lauren came over with her husband but left really quickly, and then Suzie came and did my washing-up. But then the buzzer kept on going and going.

Of course people want to see a newborn baby – but she's a newborn baby! Because she was premature I was feeling especially nervous and I wanted her to be in a calm, sterile environment.

Instead, everyone was coming off the streets with their grubby hands, which they were putting in my baby's mouth. They were waking her up, insisting they breathe their germs on her and putting their cigarette smell on her. At one time there were fourteen people in our tiny front room – and everyone seemed to have forgotten they had hands and feet as I was up and down constantly making tea and coffee for them. Even the ones that commented, 'Your stitches look really painful,' failed to help out.

In the midst of all the door-ringing my father accidentally let in a total stranger – someone who had come to deliver flowers – which upset me because I didn't want people to know where I lived. I was feeling really tired and vulnerable.

And when one girlfriend walked in with her fella, who had a stinking cold, it nearly finished me off. I sat in a ball on the sofa and refused to let anyone take Ava from me.

But what did finish me off was when I got a phone call in the evening from Gray's sister to say his parents, who had been on holiday in Spain, were coming over for a surprise visit. She said, 'Everything's sorted,' which I took to mean that they had arranged a hotel for themselves as our new flat did not have a spare room.

By 11.45 p.m. I was knackered and teary. I'd had no sleep for two days, had been up and down making cups of tea, someone with a cold had been near my precious baby, Gray and I had been squabbling about whose fault it was that we'd had all these uninvited guests and then we got 'Surprise!' from Gray's parents and his nephew. Who then wanted a ham sandwich and some tea – and who also had nowhere to sleep.

When Gray suggested his nine-year-old nephew share the bed with me while he slept on the sofa, I couldn't take it any more.

I went to the bathroom and just sobbed my heart out. Sensing my mood, Gray jumped in the car with his family and drove them around London until they could find a hotel.

The next day, Sunday, was a little better as the visitors eased off and Gray's family tidied the house and we had a big dinner with my parents. On Monday Gray shipped his family home and we had a magical day, just the three of us, sitting in bed and chilling with the flat to ourselves. I phoned the local clinic to see when the midwife might be arriving as I had begun to suspect that Ava might have a bit of jaundice. The woman at the other end of the phone was really rude – said she was far too busy to tell me when someone might be round – and referred me to another number, which turned out to be an answerphone saying, 'Do not leave a message on this number.'

On day six, Tuesday, my milk came in and I got the textbook baby blues. I was a total and utter state. I thought the world was going to end.

My boobs were as hard as ice cubes and felt like they were going to explode. And when we phoned the midwife clinic to see if they were going to come out to see us, they put the phone down on me.

I could not stop crying and feared I was suffering from postnatal depression. I had never felt so desolate and isolated and vulnerable. It wasn't me I was worried about – it was Ava. She had jaundice and now an eye infection, she was premature. I felt like she had been abandoned and I wasn't doing right by her. I felt so helpless.

The midwives only knew me as Angela Quinn and I knew that if I'd said I was Myleene Klass they would have been round a lot quicker but that made me feel even worse. Every woman should be entitled to a bit of help after she has had a baby. Your midwife is supposed to come and see you as soon as you come home from hospital but ours was putting the phone down on us.

In desperation we phoned the Lindo Wing, who told us to come back in straightaway. As soon as we got there they grabbed Ava from me to check she was OK. That made me cry even harder. Thankfully she was fine, but it upset me that Myleene Klass could do that – Angela Quinn might not have been able to.

The midwives at the Lindo were outraged that no one had been to see us and they tried calling my local unit – who also put the phone down on them. The next day Gray got on the phone. He told them he knew someone who worked for *Panorama* and he was going to come down with a camera crew. 'How dare you treat people like this,' he raged at them. It did the trick.

After a week of no midwife we now got two. But they had forgotten any scales. And then the more senior one got a chart out and decided that instead of being three weeks premature, Ava was actually three weeks late.

If it hadn't been such a tough few days I would have laughed at how this person, whose nonappearance had turned me into a miserable wreck, had got it so wrong. I felt I knew so much more than her and I'd only been Ava's mummy for a week.

22 August 2007
Gray's Diary

Both me and Leenie are used to working mad hours seven days a week. But never, ever have I been so tired. Every parent I know told me — but I have to say I didn't believe them. Well, I was wrong. Big time. I'm bloody knackered. Can't believe how tiring it is. All night we are awake. No one tells you the noises babies make while they are sleeping. And if they go quiet you will be checking they're still breathing every two minutes. Sleep was a part of your old life — say goodbye to it for the next couple of years — and who knows, by then baby number two might be coming along.

It's hard work. But trust me, it's the best feeling in the world when you hold your baby or look into her eyes. This is what life is really about and not the other rubbish we worry about every day — the house, the cars, money, work. Your new baby is priceless and you will love them more than you ever thought you could love. You would give them your last drop of blood.

I can't remember what it was like before Ava and I don't want to. Other parents have told me I would only get what life is about when it happened to me and now it has I fully understand what they mean. Mothers are a great thing, I have so much respect for you all and what you go through, especially my girl for giving me baby Ava. I'm so proud of you and how great a mama you are already.

September 2007
Epilogue

It's only been a month but now I can barely remember my pregnancy, let alone life without Ava.

My world has become a routine of feeding, changing, sleep, putting a wash on, feeding, changing, sleep, putting a wash on . . . I have become one of those women who leaves home without brushing her hair or cleaning her teeth. It takes me two hours to get out of the flat and my last good sleep was the two hours I had during labour. Outside of looking after Ava, I struggle to do one thing a day.

But I wouldn't have it any other way.

I have become a different person and I know that I won't ever be the Myleene I was before. Pregnancy changed me, but that was mainly the hormones. Now I am a mummy I have changed again.

I cry more and I empathise more. Stories of children being harmed make me howl. I love being part of the mummy's club where I can talk about labour and stitches and baby poo. I have lots and lots of conversations about baby poo.

I am obsessed with my daughter. Gray calls me 'stalker mummy' because I sit and stare at her for hours. Every noise and facial expression she makes fascinates me. I never knew I could be so happy just being at home with my baby. If I'd known how wonderful it was, I would have started having children years ago.

Gray knows that my love for Ava surpasses anything I have ever known. He is OK about it because he feels the same. When he said to me one evening, 'I love you, but I LOVE her,' I understood. It is love that comes from the pit of my stomach. It is totally unconditional.

I thought I would be desperate to go back to work but, although I started doing a few hours of work a month after she was born, it was an utter wrench leaving her.

Gray had to take me away from her in stages. First twenty minutes, then a couple of hours. I couldn't believe how difficult I found it without her and I was constantly worried.

I still preferred to have her with me and there have already been times she has breast-fed on me – yes, I'm still breast-feeding – while I presented my radio show, at photoshoots and at restaurant meetings. I take pashminas with me everywhere.

Ava has made contract signing a little more interesting after she projectile vomited in the office of my very posh lawyer.

But I also realised that my plans of having her with me all the time, and not having any routine in her life, might not be fair on her. I have always wanted to be a working mum but I never realised the guilt that would come with it – you want the best of both worlds. To be honest, I'm still trying to work things out.

I realise now that worry will never truly leave me, just like it has never left my parents.

I worry about whether she is too hot or too cold, whether she's comfortable, whether she's ill or dehydrated, whether she's still breathing, whether she's hungry or got wind, whether I should wake her up or let her sleep in a dirty nappy.

Every squeak she makes at night has me running to her. The first time she was sick I was in floods of tears, wanting desperately to be ill in her place.

I have put a lot of pressure on myself to be the perfect mother but I have learned that all my friends were right when they told me there is no such thing. You can only do your best.

Becoming parents has changed my relationship with Gray. I can't understand all those couples who have 'band aid' babies to mend their broken relationships. Having a baby is hard on a couple – even one as close as Gray and me.

The whirlwind that came into our lives and shook it to the core came as a shock to us.

The sleep deprivation, in particular, makes everything seem worse. We both really did think we would be the exception to the rule but within just a few days we were both so exhausted that we were snapping at each other.

I felt resentful towards Gray because he went out 'wetting the baby's head'. He felt resentful towards me, feeling I was 'hogging' Ava and not trusting him to look after her.

We have got through it by constantly talking to each other and communicating. We have reminded each other that it was us first, before Ava came along. And we have also become closer and more in love because we are now a family, we are knitted together for eternity.

We are already talking about when we are going to start trying for baby number two . . .

Glossary

Amniotic fluid: Clear waters surrounding the baby in the amniotic sac. It cushions the baby and protects it from infection.

Antenatal: Before the delivery of the baby.

Baby blues: A mild depression which many women experience in the first few days after giving birth.

Braxton Hicks: Irregular contractions which can occur throughout pregnancy.

Cervix: The lower end of the uterus which leads to the vagina. It gradually opens (dilates) during labour.

Embryo: An early foetus before it resembles a human.

Epidural: A local anaesthetic that is injected into the space between your spinal column and spinal cord, numbing the nerves to the lower part of the body.

Foetus: The name given to a baby in the womb after eight weeks of development.

Gestation: The period of time given from the date of the first day of the last period to delivery. Full-term gestation is between 38 and 42 weeks.

Latch on: The correct position for the baby to be in when feeding from the breast – the baby should have its mouth open wide and not just sucking at the nipple.

Ovaries: The sex glands which produce key female hormones and eggs. There is one either side of the uterus.

Ovulation: The optimum time for conception when a mature egg is released from the ovaries.

Placenta: Organ responsible for providing nutrients to the foetus and expelling its waste products. It is delivered after the birth.

Postnatal: Mother and baby after the birth.

Show: Sticky pink mucus which plugs the womb during pregnancy but comes out of the vagina at the start of labour.

TENS machine: A method of pain relief in which electric pads are placed on the back discharging a stimulus that interferes with the pain signals to the brain.

Umbilical cord: Tube which carries oxygen and nourishment from the placenta to the baby. The cord is cut after the delivery – leaving a stump which will fall off after a few days, revealing the belly button.

Uterus/womb: Pear-shaped organ in the abdomen where the embryo develops.

My recommended beauty tips

Pregnancy can be so exhausting that it can be easy to forgot beauty routines for an extra five minutes' sleep. There are also lots of creams and treatments that you can no longer use.

But I kept on my exfoliating as I am mad about it. And I became obsessed with slicking myself with oil to prevent any stretch marks.

I started with Bio-Oil then I used the Clarins Body Treatment Oil but my favourite was Burt's Bees' Mama Bee Nourishing Baby Oil, which was phenomenal because it smelled of lemon and almond. I felt like I smelled good enough to eat.

I also went to the health-food store and got pure vitamin E oil and I rubbed it into all the places where I was most likely to get stretch marks.

I didn't get a single stretch mark – although I can't tell you whether that was down to good genes or slathering up like an oil slick. But who wants to take the chance!

My recommended books

Pregnancy Questions & Answers: Everything you need to know, trimester by trimester by the editors and experts at BabyCentre. co.uk: I really enjoyed this book because it presented all the medical stuff in easy-to-read bullet points. I especially enjoyed their week-by-week account of what is happening to you and your baby, which I also got sent to me via their weekly email. Very informative, but not so good on the emotional aspects.

What To Expect When You're Expecting and *What To Expect The First Year* by Heidi E. Murkoff, Arlene Eisenberg and Sandee E. Hathaway: One book for your pregnancy and one for the first year of your baby's life, these are the bibles of the baby world – full of facts and information about everything you need to know.

The Yummy Mummy's Survival Guide: How To Put The Mmmm Back Into Motherhood by Liz Fraser: I really enjoyed the humour in this until I read her bit about how she suffered from bulimia and carried on making herself sick during her pregnancies. I admired her honesty but I had to put the book down after that because I realised I had nothing in common with her.

Pregnancy Companion by Dr John C. Anderson, Dr Tom Boogert, Dr Greg J. Kesby, Dr Andrew C. McLennan, Ms Janette O'Connor, Dr Robert D. Robertson, Dr Fergus P. Scott: A good week-by-week guide with room for you to add notes about your own growth.

The New Contented Little Baby Book by Gina Ford: Worth a look even if it is just so you can know what the big Gina Ford debate is about. A good reference point because she does come up with some ideas worth following, but her routines were too regimented for me.

The Complete Book of Baby Names Traditional and Modern by Hilary Spence: It's fun flicking through all the weird and obscure names and this had thousands to choose from. We found Bailey in it.

My recommended clothes shops

I was lucky because it was the season of maxi dresses and smock dresses so I got lots of non-maternity clothes in bigger sizes. But the best maternity ranges were:

Marks & Spencer – they sent me a shedload of their maternity clothes and their normal clothes in bigger sizes. I can't thank them enough.

Crave maternity (www.cravematernity.co.uk): These are on the internet and had some good casual bits.

Isabella Oliver (www.isabellaoliver.com): A slightly more upmarket maternity dress shop which had some great outfits for nights out.

Thank yous

Nicole Lampert. Writing this book with you has been such a brilliant experience. Thanks for guiding me through the wonderful world of muslins, swaddling and circular blankets! As I've said before, you are an inspirational working mummy and I know this is the start of a long, wonderful friendship. Any woman who sends a mummy in need a breast pump in the post is a friend for life in my books! Big x for Benjy.

FAMILY... Gray. I watch you and our beautiful baby sleeping beside me and I can't help but thank God for sending you both to me. You always said this would be an amazing journey and now we have another passenger with us. I love you more and more every day. Panda x

(Grand) Dad and Lola, for being the most amazing grandparents to Ava and for being there to help and love us all.

My sister Chez and brother Don and Jake and M. I know you will be there for her whenever she or I need you and that's what counts.

Cousin John. Glamour, fashion, shoes and handbags. She's in your hands now!

Lisa Duffy. For being so wise, so kind and a big sister to me. You have helped when others didn't know how to. Love you x

Nana Ita and Grandpa Willie. Thank you for helping me, Ita, throughout my pregnancy and understanding what I was going through. You were unbelievable and helped me when I really needed a friend. Proud to be your daughter-in-law.

FRIENDS... Andrea Kyriacou. Wherever would I be without you?! You have always looked out for me and continue to do so. How you find time for everyone, I will never know. Superwoman has nothing on you girly! Love you dearly.

Betty Gat at babysafe. Thank you for teaching us such vital skills. I only hope I never have to use them!

Carryl Thomas. You seem to constantly have time for everyone and the kindest, calmest serenity about you. You are a fantastic example of what a yummy mummy is all about. Big x to handsome godson Joel.

Clare and Joshy. From college days to motherhood! Thank you for being on the end of the phone, keeping me sane and reassuring me that I am in fact perfectly normal. Either that, or you're just as mad as me!

Claudine Tindall and Sienna. For teaching me that hiccups aren't the end of the world, that mummies are each other's best friends and that you are one in a million and I'm so lucky to have you.

Jaqui Press and Lauren. You constantly amaze me with your sheer determination and endurance in the face of adversity. You are an inspirational, lovely lady.

Mel and Mena. You have been a true, true friend. I will never forget the day you came over, cleaned my kitchen, bought me a chicken (not bad for a veggie!) and showed me that friends are worth their weight in gold. You are a remarkable woman and I adore you. Thank you for our chats and your friendship.

Uncle Donald and Nathan 'bear cub'.

Lauren Laverne and Bean. We have been through so much. I'm so glad that we had the chance to go on this journey together. It has been all the richer with you by my side and I look forward to the day Fergus, Ava, you and I sit in our gardens eating ice cream. Namely as it means our houses will be finished! You're the bestest friend I could ever have wished for.

Jill Kenton and Rachel. A remarkable kind friend with a heart as big as her smile. Thanks for being there, for providing the humour and showing me such kindness.

Jo Tutchener Fox. For trying to help keep this mummy yummy with all your lovely products! Can't wait to be your neighbour and for Ava to have pink things and a cat to play with!

Uncle Jonathan Shalit. Whatever would we do without you? You've been a constant support, inspiration and friend to my little family. You've changed my life for which I am eternally grateful. Thank you for everything you've done for us. Just remember, I'm counting on you to introduce Ava to fishcakes at the Ivy!

Julie Armstrong. You have certainly put the humour into this whole experience! Your honesty and down-to-earth approach have helped me no end. Thank you for being the biggest mummy ever! Big x to my stunning goddaughter, Layla Brooke.

Katie Birtwistle.

Soren 'Gurden' Johansen. The three musketeers have just recruited a new member to the tightest gang in the world. Few people can ever say they can rely on a person one hundred per cent, but that is true of you.

Suzie Shaw. We have been through everything together, and now here we are mummies! I love you always and having Ava now has taught me what a resilient, strong woman you really are. To have gone through everything you did alone, I salute you. Love my best gal and my gorgeous godson Corey. And for being my confidant, thank you. Now hurry up and have babies!

Mandy and Nichola Barham. Maria Malone. Michelle and Andrew.

MEDICAL . . . Peter Mason. The most charming man that ever walked the earth! For your guidance, strength, kindness and, most importantly, for delivering my 'princess' to me, thank you from the bottom of my heart.

Maxine at Peter Masons.

Sharon French, my incredible midwife, and everyone at the Lindo wing.

WORK . . . Leila Martyn, for the midnight phone calls, and for always knowing the right things to say.

Severine Berman. You are a one-woman dynamo! I thank you heart and soul for our chats, your honesty, your perseverance when I've literally forgotten what day it is, and for being such a unique and genuine friend to me and Ava bear. We absolutely adore you. You hurry up and have fabulous big-haired babies too!

Lea, Richy Rich and Laura from Shalit Global.

Uncle Simon Jones and Shane. Thank you to the loveliest uncles in the world! If you look after Ava the way you do her mama then she is without a doubt one lucky girl. Thank you for your friendship, ever constant honesty and superb 'Boney M' dancing skills!

Everyone at Hackford Jones.

Ali Gunn, Carolyn Thorne, Gareth Fletcher, KT Forster and everyone at Virgin for all your hard work and for making this book a reality.

John Stewart and everyone at Myleeneklass.co.uk.

THE FANS . . . To everyone who thought of me and my family throughout and after my pregnancy, I thank you. I have never received so many cards, gifts, toys and well wishes. I am so lucky to have such incredible support from such dedicated and kind people. On behalf of Ava, Gray and myself, thanks to you all. And if you're pregnant, congratulations. I hope this book makes you feel somewhat reassured!

Index

MK denotes Myleene Klass.